# Rave Reviews for
## *Create the Vitality You Crave*

"*Create the Vitality You Crave* is more than a book; it is a companion for anyone on the path to wellness. Lori Finlay doesn't just present information; she equips you with the tools to transform that knowledge into a sustainable lifestyle of health and vitality. Her book is a testament to the power of integrating body, mind, and spirit in the healing process, and I highly recommend it to anyone seeking a comprehensive guide to becoming their best self."

*Kirsten, P., UT*

"*Create the Vitality You Crave* is a fantastic reference and read for anyone interested in living a more vibrant life. As a health coach and yoga instructor I would recommend this book to someone just beginning to make positive changes in their health as well as anyone already familiar with the wellness world and everyone in between. This book is engaging with many personal stories and examples, science backed research, motivating information on habits and applying the information. I will definitely be recommending this book to clients and friends who are wondering where to begin or what next step to take in improving their health."

*Kim N., CA*

"The book covers a wide range of topics including nutrition, exercise, mental health, and self-care practices. It offers evidence-based advice interwoven with personal anecdotes and practical tips, making the content relatable and actionable. The narrative is both informative and engaging, with a tone that is encouraging and supportive rather than prescriptive.

   *Create the Vitality You Crave* is a valuable resource for any woman seeking to enhance her overall well-being. Its balanced approach, epitomized by the floors and ceilings concept, provides a sustainable framework for personal growth. This book is a must-read for those looking to embrace a healthier, more vibrant life with realistic and achievable goals."

*Laura K., NV*

"*Create the Vitality You Crave: Epigenetics 101 to Unlock Your Healing Powers* by Lori Finlay, is a comprehensive guide to achieving a happier and healthier life by understanding and leveraging the principles of epigenetics. Authored with a blend of scientific insight and practical wisdom, this book offers readers a roadmap from A to Z, covering essential aspects vital for optimal well-being.

Furthermore, it delves into the importance of hormones with remarkable depth. It helps readers make informed choices to fuel their bodies optimally. The book highlights the importance of understanding hormonal balance, especially as we age, offering strategies to support hormonal health naturally."

*Russ. K., NV*

"My experience as a psychotherapist over the years has caused me to appreciate the essential connection between our minds and our bodies. In this book, Lori has eloquently described this connection with excellent support from evidence-based scientific research. I also appreciate the personal and relatable information she shares and believe that many women will identify with her stories.

In this compelling and inspiring book, Lori shares the secrets she has uncovered on her quest for heath and wellness. Lori's personal examples illustrate how she has defied her own genetic predispositions and family history. Any reader will be inspired by the knowledge and wisdom she has accumulated over the years!"

*Joanna K., GA*

"This book is truly life changing, even lifesaving and most significantly life lifting. Vitality is the perfect word for this work that encompasses total health. This book is a comprehensive guide in navigating women's health.

It reads like a letter from your best friend, experienced sister, and knowledgeable medical team all in one. A resource you can trust and come back to again and again.

The research and science aspects were delivered clearly in a way my non science disposition was easily able to comprehend with insights for practical application."

*Jennie M., NC*

*I am humbled and grateful for these reviews!! As a Solopreneur, the success of my book comes from word of mouth and reviews. I would be so grateful if you could write a review so that others will be notified of this priceless life-transforming information.*

*Sincerely,*
*Lori Finlay*

# CREATE THE

## Vitality

## YOU CRAVE

Epigenetics 101 to
Unlock Your Healing Power

LORI FINLAY
MSN, NP, CNS, BCC

The author of this book does not dispense medical advice or prescribe the use of any technique as a form of treatment for physical, emotional, or medical problems without the advice of a physician, either directly or indirectly. The intent of the author is only to offer information of a general nature to help you in your quest for spiritual, emotional, mental, and physical well-being. In the event you use any of the information in this book for yourself, the author assumes no responsibility for your actions.

To protect the privacy of others, certain names and details have been changed.

ISBN: 979-8-9909102-2-5 (Hardcover)
ISBN: 979-8-218-36603-2 (Paperback)
ISBN: 979-8-9909102-0-1 (Ebook)
ISBN: 979-8-9909102-1-8 (Audiobook)

HEALTH & FITNESS / Women's Health
HEALTH & FITNESS / Longevity
HEALTH & FITNESS / Alternative Therapies

Book Design by Michelle M. White
Cover art derived from illustration by Elymas at Stock.Adobe.com

Printed in the United States of America

1st edition, September 2024

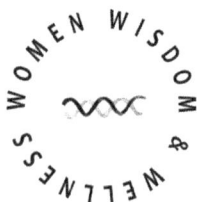

WOMEN WISDOM & WELLNESS

# Contents

## SECTION 8

### *Closing Thoughts*

# Acknowledgments

As I reflect on the journey that led to the creation of this book, I am humbled by the intricate tapestry of support, love, and divine guidance that has woven itself into every word on these pages. Of the five love languages, as coined by Gary Chapman, words of affirmation or acknowledgement are right up there for me. Thus, this list of acknowledgments may be longer than most.

First and foremost, to my Father in Heaven, Jesus Christ, and the Holy Ghost—your constant companionship and guiding light continue to transform me and my life. You are whom I have trusted to co-create this book and my life. You are my compass, my rock, and the unwavering anchor that steadies me through every day and night.

To my cherished big brother, hero, and confidant Barry—your unwavering support carried me through my most challenging of days and nights. Your love, encouragement, extraordinary support, wisdom, and daily check-ins have been the steady heartbeat that has propelled me forward, even in moments of doubt or trial.

To my precious grandchildren—your boundless joy and unbridled wonder have reignited the childlike magic within me. The arm wrestles, planks, pillow fights, hiking, crawling through snow caves, water sports, dancing, or playing for hours were the reward for regaining my own vitality, inspiring me to empower others to regain theirs. You have been a reminder of the beauty that graces our world, filling my days with laughter and my heart with warmth beyond my wildest imagination.

To my nieces and nephews—who have showered me with unconditional love and cheered me on for years. Chillin' with you, your laughter, and love have been a profound source of boundless joy and fulfillment. The precious moments we have shared have fueled me, reminding me of the profound impact that love and encouragement can have on one's heart and soul.

To my surrogate families, the Olives and the Wilcox gang—your embrace has been a sanctuary of love and acceptance. You have filled emptiness and brought bounteous love. Each of you has left an indelible mark on my heart, filling my life with warmth, laughter, and a sense of belonging that I will forever cherish.

To my beloved friends, Brenda Yates, Anna Marshall Powers, Joanna Goulding Kestor, Bobbi Horne, Diann Harries, Michelle Marchant-Johnson, Candy Wright, and the Women of Christ—your friendship and sisterhood have been a beacon of light in my life. You have helped me to find my authentic voice and to own my power. In your company, I have found strength, courage, and incredible encouragement that have sustained me and propelled me forward in my own re*creation* journey.

To the healers, Dr. Melodie Billiot, Dr. Nelli Biddix, Dr. Russell Friedman, Dr. Erika Bradshaw, Joel Crosby, and Emily Stovall—your brilliant minds, healing touch, attentive listening, extraordinary intuition, and compassionate presence have been a source of solace and renewal. Your gifts have helped me heal in ways I could only dream of. You are the ones that helped restore the vitality that I craved. I am in deep gratitude.

To the courageous women who have accompanied me in my journey of recovery—your strength, vulnerability, and courage have been transformational. Together, we've shared tears, laughter, and triumphs, forging bonds that have enriched my life beyond measure. Thank you for your authenticity, your spiritual strength, wisdom, and your enduring friendship.

To my mentors, Dr. Kyrin Dunston, Dr. Anna Cabeca, and Carol Tuttle—your wisdom and guidance have lit a fire within and given me permission to go for it. You have been a source of inspiration driving me to reach for the stars and embrace my true purpose.

To Sarah Grace Allred and the women of the Alliance—your unfaltering encouragement, vision of my potential, and camaraderie have been a source of inspiration and empowerment. In your presence, I have found a tribe of kindred spirits who have lifted me up and encouraged me to let my light shine.

To my coaches and counselors, Brooke Snow, Crystal Hollenbeck, Tony Overbay, Sandra Brown, Nikki Eisenhauer, and Benita Esposito—your compassion, empathy, and consistent advocacy have been the cornerstone of my healing journey. Your guidance has helped me navigate the depths of my soul with courage and grace, allowing me to emerge stronger and more resilient than ever before.

To my amazing clients who have walked alongside me in my expansive career—your trust, vulnerability, and resilience have taught me invaluable lessons about healing and what it truly means to be a healer. Each of you has left an indelible mark on my journey, and I am forever grateful for the privilege of accompanying you on your path to wellness.

And finally, I offer deep gratitude for my amazing friend and editor, Lauren Johnson—your dedication, incredible patience, and keen insight have transformed these words into a symphony of wisdom and authenticity. Your unwavering commitment to excellence has elevated this work to heights I never thought possible. Together, may we bless many with the gift of vitality!

*With a heart overflowing with love and gratitude,*
*Lori*

# Introduction

*When Health is absent, Wisdom cannot reveal itself;*
*Art cannot manifest; Strength cannot be exerted;*
*Wisdom is useless, and Reason is powerless.*
~ARDOMORE HEROPHILUS, 30 B.C. FATHER OF ANATOMY

In the summer of 2022, when I was midway through composing this book, my husband of 22 years called me long distance during what was supposed to be a short trip to Massachusetts and told me he was filing for divorce. To make the shocking scenario even worse, he actually delivered the message by reading—word for word—a letter he had written. It wasn't a conversation. There was no apology or empathy. This phone call happened shortly after we had moved from Atlanta to Tampa, Florida, and remodeled our home to prepare for our new life of retirement. He was finalizing his last week of work in Atlanta, with retirement parties planned to celebrate our new life that was about to unfold.

Not only was I mentally and emotionally flabbergasted, but my body had its own reaction, and my spirit was crushed. In the weeks and months that followed, I needed to rally all my years of training about what restorative self-care and functional medicine really meant if I wanted to survive, let alone thrive!

I was in awe of what my body went through as I prepared for divorce, with all the legal maneuvering and challenges my ex-husband put me through at an amplified pace. Sleep became elusive and fears for my future engrossed me as I was forced to start life all over again at age 62, with my full-time career in nursing 20 years behind me. The principles I teach in this book got me through this challenging time, which makes me one of the lucky ones. Research[1] has shown that women who go through a *betrayal* trauma—whether from abuse, grief, loss, death, or divorce—will develop breast cancer at least two to three times the rate of other women within two years of the trauma.

I knew that. And I knew it was imperative that I do everything in my power to keep my body, mind, and spirit resonating at the highest level possible during the process to follow. I didn't want to join that betrayal trauma statistic. Even though I already had solid self-care rituals in place, ate nutritious whole foods, and exercised regularly, I knew I needed to upgrade everything about my health in order to come out with enduring vitality. I knew that some things had to go (whether hopes, dreams, resentments, anger, food, or furniture), or at least be relegated to the back burner, to allow even more time for me to take care of my wounded self.

As a former Clinical Nurse Specialist and Nurse Practitioner who has studied Functional Medicine extensively and embraced the new science of Epigenetics in pursuit of my own health and wellness, I have found that addressing my spiritual journey has been a mandatory part of whole healing. Regardless of *your* belief system or faith, I recommend that you connect to your Higher Power, Spirit, Universe, Divinity, Source, or whatever entity you choose for true healing. Aligning with God or our Higher Power is where we can amplify our lives and healing powers.

Personally, I'm a devoted Christian woman, and I love the word of God. For me, Co-Creating with Christ each and every day is what got me through the toughest of tough times. I feel, and we are taught in 12-step recovery work, that we are limited by relying solely on our *own* power. Thus, in the pages that follow, you will see scriptures quoted occasionally, right along with scientists and health experts.

## My Hope and Prayer

If you are fatigued, feeling unwell, off-balance, and tired of being blown-off by the conventional medical system when you need help, my hope is that delving into my words will provide insight, bring clarity, and help you discover all the ways you can *amplify your power* to regain your vitality! In the pages ahead, I've sorted, synthesized, and summarized years of study that I've used to not only regain and restore my own health, but for the health of my clients as well. Included is substantial information you can use to claim your power of healing, move forward, and improve *your* health at a cellular level.

This book is being published about two years after that fated phone call, yet I believe that all things will be redeemed, and all things happen in right timing. I hope that this is the right timing for you, too. The healing practices detailed herein not only kept me going but provided the hope and healing that have catapulted me into this new chapter of my life.

I want to help women in their 30s and 40s understand *and* listen to their bodies, so they don't inadvertently do what I did to mine when I was that age. I also want to help the women in mid-life who may be dealing with the results of neglected self-care and health. If you're ready to *finally* own *your* healing powers and create vitality, then this book is for you. With a little education and a dose of inspiration, you can achieve the vitality you crave to be the woman, wife, mother, leader, "girlboss," or whatever role you may wish to express.

It's time for you to *Create the Vitality You Crave.*

# Section 1

## Challenging the Norms of Modern Sickness Medicine

# One

## Self-care Isn't Selfish

*"Self-care is how you take your power back."*
~Lalah Delia

Both women, and the men they love, tend to put off self-care until their bodies are screaming, but for different reasons. Women were divinely designed to be nurturers and to have diffuse awareness (or multi-focus), able to assess and focus on the needs of everyone around them. This often means women put their needs on the backburner, fearing that self-care is selfish, or simply feeling there isn't enough time.

Men, on the other hand, are single focused. They were divinely designed to completely ignore a stubbed or bleeding toe if they were out chasing after a woolly mammoth to provide for or protect their family. As a result, their symptoms could be screaming at them long before they even notice or allow themselves to take the time to find out what is causing the pain. They grow accustomed to their insidious symptoms.

As a professional woman for years, I was dealing with both yin and yang energies. While I was using yin feminine energy caring for patients all day, I was also in significant yang energy working long hours at Mach 1 speeds, which the female body is not designed for. Not only was I exhausted from the long work hours, but I was also getting only three to five hours of sleep a night due to a severe sleeping disorder. I kept pushing myself through.

I was exhausted! I didn't realize how bad it was until I did a sleep study a few years later. It took me that long to cry uncle and get some help. My sleep study revealed that of the eight hours I was in bed, I slept for only three hours, but had 78 arousals. And I don't mean the good kind, either.

At age 40, I got married, moved across the country, and became a stepmom to teens. Even though some of this was Eustress (the good kind), it was still stress. By the time I was 42, my body had had enough, and I crashed. I had ignored the signs and symptoms for so long that my body was nearly shut down.

By the time I "hit the wall," I was in premature ovarian failure (premature menopause). My adrenals were nearly flat lined. I had to take a prescription for cortisol (Cortef) because my adrenals could barely function. The fatigue was excruciating! I could accomplish about two hours of productivity, but only after napping for two hours. My days were up and down and up and down. I could not make it through my church meetings and then come home and make dinner for my family, so I had to choose one or the other. I was struggling to even cope, yet alone be my best self for my new husband and family.

While I had incredible education and knowledge as a Clinical Nurse Specialist in Critical Care and Adult Nurse Practitioner, I was a specialist in what I call "sickness medicine,"—that is, healing those with acute illness or life-threatening situations. I was clueless about really "healing" the body, just as I was clueless about the symptoms that I was experiencing. I didn't know that my adverse childhood events (ACEs) or unhealed betrayal traumas were contributing to the vicious cycle of endless proving and disproving that kept me running ragged. Although I was eating a healthier diet than 90% of Americans, having worked in cardiology for years and witnessing the fallout of poor diets, I had no idea that my mental and physical stress and sleep-deprived lifestyle were wreaking havoc on my body and my genes—from skin to skeleton.

Self-care was out of the question. I was too busy.

When I could ignore my symptoms no longer and sought medical help, I was dismissed, disrespected, gaslit, and shamed by my colleagues. An endocrinologist literally told me, "There's nothing wrong. Your labs are all within normal limits. This is all in your head." I imagine that you've been told something similar when faced with crushing symptoms and no diagnosis or cure, whether by a medical professional or a well-meaning friend. When a former colleague asked me, "How much time do you spend researching your sickness on the internet?" and I offered a muted response, he patted me on the knee and said, "You should just leave your healthcare up to me." Two days later he tried to prescribe hormones based on false positive lab data, which I had to point out to him. I promptly "fired" him. After those troubling back-to-back encounters, I thought, *if I'm going through this, with all of my education and the ability to talk the lingo, what on earth are my girlfriends dealing with when they see their healthcare providers?* I knew I had to make a difference, but first I needed to heal myself! I had to take care of myself. I had to be my own health advocate.

And you do, too.

In my work with clients and among my friends and family, I see women who are exhausted. Depleted. Wiped out emotionally, physically, spiritually, and mentally. Wiped out to the point that they are hanging on with their fingernails in almost every role. Additionally, they are struggling in relationships; they are struggling in their families and in their roles as mothers—unsure if they can even do this anymore. For those that are working outside the home, they are struggling there, too! As a result, for most women, expressing their divine spiritual gifts is way out of reach as well.

This kind of struggle requires more than just standing tall and continuing to push through whatever comes before you while straightening your crown. You must practice self-care in order to be your best self for *yourself* as well as those you care about. Unaddressed physiological challenges are sabotaging women's attempts to stand up straight, to cope, and to "keep on, keeping on."

Sadly, most women do *not* realize that they have a physiological reason for feeling so horrible. Instead, they try to "fix" it in ways that don't solve the underlying problem. In fact, they take on even *more*. They go to the gym and bust their butt to lose weight, with no success. They work with other coaches that encourage and teach them some "tools" to help them change—to no avail. They go see their doctor and get a pill for an ill, never getting to the root cause of what is really going on.

Let's get real. Right now, on a scale of 1 to 5 (1 being "not a chance" and 5 being "absolutely"), how confident are you that, at the age of 65, you will have the energy to take your grandkids to Disney World for the day? What about traveling the world with your soulmate? What about having the mental clarity, passion, and drive to continue to make a huge contribution in the world? How confident are you that you will look and feel sexy and have a passionate sex life with amazing orgasms? If you're like the majority of my clients and others who I talk with, I'll bet you have a lot of answers ranging from 1 to 3, if you're lucky.

If those goals and desires don't even sound like remote possibilities from where you are right now, then this book will show you the way so you can heal and create this future.

What if I said you *can* regain your vitality? What if I said you *can* straighten your crown and feel tall, energized, witty, happy, and serene again? What if I said you *can* have the passion and vitality described above? I know first-hand it's possible, because that is how I feel today! Today at 64, I'm healthier, happier, stronger, and more svelte than I was at 44. I enjoy competing with 30- and 40-year-olds on my Peloton, advanced Pilates, strength training, kayaking, the Hydrofoil surfboard, and all kinds of activity and adventure.

You do *not* have to be a victim to feeling unwell. You don't have to be a victim of your inherited genes, Big Western Medicine, Big Pharma, or Big Food! Read on to find out more.

## *Consider This*

- *What symptoms are you experiencing right now? List them all, considering how you feel spiritually, emotionally, mentally, and physically.*

- *What self-care activities would you love to do if time or money were not a factor?*

*Two*

# Dysfunctional Versus Functional Medicine

*"The doctor of the future will give no medicines,*
*but will interest his patients in the care of the human frame,*
*in diet, and in the causes and prevention of disease."*
~Thomas Edison

In *Metabolical—The Lure and the Lies of Processed Food, Nutrition, and Modern Medicine*,[1] Robert Lustig, MD, retired pediatric endocrinologist, clearly outlines the "diabolical" nature of the intertwined medical industries and why they are all profiting from so many chronic health conditions.

Dr. Lustig explains that "The US has the best doctors, hospitals, medical technologies, the most innovative procedures, best and newest drugs, yet we spend the most per capita on *healthcare* (*italics added*) than any country in the world!" Unfortunately, American's have the *worst health outcomes* of any country in the Organization for Economic Co-operation and Development (OECD), which includes 37 of the richest countries.

Hmmm, what's going on here?

## Our Dysfunctional System

We spend 97.5 % of our healthcare budget on *treatment* and only 2.5% on *prevention*. Not a big bang for the buck, given that we have such egregious outcomes for the amount of money spent.

Personally, I call this "sickcare." Don't get me wrong—if I were hit by a car or had a major health issue, I would want our Western doctors to help with such an acute situation. However, there is so much more that we can do ourselves to *prevent* disease so that we don't have to rely on doctors in the future. There are so many things we can do so we are not victims to our family medical history or our current lifestyle choices or our doctor's edicts. Otherwise, we will continue to suffer the consequences of our daily/current lifestyle choices, and those consequences will only become worse.

## Unequal treatment of women

It is still prevalent for women to be victimized by the system of dysfunctional, corporate healthcare that is Big Medicine and Big Pharma. Women continue to experience "medical gaslighting" scenarios in doctors' offices across the country.

I worked with a 30-year-old woman who, after presenting to a doctor with a myriad of symptoms that made her feel "old," was told, "Well, of course you feel old. You're 30." To that I say, WHAT? She was a 30-year-old former athlete, yet the endocrinologist sent her out the door with a synthetic thyroid prescription without doing any other diagnostic testing. That was a 15-minute doc in the box, dysfunctional, and corporate medicine approach. They simply checked off the CPT billing codes, gave her the bill, prescribed a synthetic pill, then sent her out the door. With Functional Medicine, seeking for the root cause approach, I uncovered her heavy metal toxicity, Epstein Barre, and significant hormonal imbalances. This is why she felt "old."

In my opinion, she was a victim of Western medicine.

I was, too.

When I went to the doctor with severe restless leg syndrome, I was told "it's all in your head." But what I didn't know and professionals didn't help with, was that I had severe, heavy metal toxicity in my body that was impacting my sleep and causing my restless leg syndrome—*not* my thoughts. Instead of testing or even considering me for heavy metals, the doctor put me on an addictive drug (a long-acting Benzodiazepine, similar to Valium) and said, "You'll be on this the rest of your life, and your dose will most likely get higher and higher." I was victimized by that medical "assessment." It took me eight years to get off that drug, and I was only able to do so after finding another medical practitioner—a chiropractor—to help me diagnose and heal the heavy metal toxicity in my body.

About a year later, when I was experiencing severe fatigue, I went to an endocrinologist, who told me my adrenals were fine. He knew nothing of heavy metal toxicity either, thus he did not test for it. When I removed the terrible silver amalgam (toxic mercury) fillings out of my mouth, I thought I'd get better. However, when my white blood cell count was severely low, my Functional Health doctor found Epstein Barre. That's another reason I felt so fatigued, but it wasn't until 10 years later that I finally found the black mold in my body. And it wasn't until after getting DNA testing years later, that the common denominator of my symptoms was revealed—*poor Glutathione detox pathways!* I'll talk about the magic of Glutathione later in Chapters 8 and 11 and why it's so important for you to consider in your vitality journey.

## Clinical trial disparities

It's more than during office visits that women are gaslit and in-validated for their symptoms. There continues to be significant disparity in clinical trials, with women being underrepresented across the board. Women have been excluded from clinical studies for decades, in part due to menstrual cycles and changes in the female body. But I think those are exactly the reasons why women's bodies *should* be studied!

If you examine clinical studies, in any category, whether they're about nutrition, health, physical fitness, cardiology, or hematology, etc., you will find that these studies are usually about middle-aged or young fit men—*not* about women. As such, they don't present the real facts.

Unfortunately, women and medical providers have found that even *if* a study is designed and focuses entirely on women and women's health issues, the motive may *not* be focused on improving women's health. One example is the Women's Health Initiative (WHI) study, with a whopping price tag of over one billion dollars, which enrolled 160,000 American women and lasted from 1991 to 2005. We were told that the study was designed to examine if Hormone Replacement Therapy (HRT) was associated with risk reduction or preventing heart disease, breast and colorectal cancer, and osteoporosis in postmenopausal women. The medical world was shocked when headlines in *The New York Times*, the BBC, and JAMA (the *Journal of American Medical Association*) all stated that the study "was stopped not only because HRT increased breast cancer risk, but also because of increased risks of coronary artery disease, stroke and pulmonary embolism." As a result of this news, HRT usage dropped by 70 percent around the world, and women were now left suffering through the symptoms of menopause without support.

Unfortunately, despite the one-billion-dollar price tag, the WHI was poorly designed and had significant flaws. First, the women were a much older population, starting HRT at the age of 60 to 69, which is considered at least a decade past the start time for optimal benefit. They were also a very unhealthy population, with over 20 percent obese, 35 percent considered overweight, nearly 36 percent being treated for hypertension (HTN), or high blood pressure, and nearly half were current or past smokers.

Additionally, the drugs used in the WHI were *synthetic* hormones, not *bioidentical*. Premarin is a conjugated equine estrogen made from **Pre**gnant **Mar**e Ur**in**e—thus Premarin. Additionally, the study used synthetic progesterone called progestins. It has been shown that it's the progestins or *synthetic* progesterone that causes breast cancer.[2,3,4,5]

Women and their providers were all left with the notion that *all* hormones were bad, when clearly bioidentical hormones are safer and even preventative.

Now, let me address some ugly details behind the design and objective of the WHI study.

Jacques Rossouw, a cardiologist, was one of the chief investigators of the WHI. Dr. Rossouw clearly stated that his goal was to "shake up the medical establishment and change the thinking about hormones."[6] And, he and his buddies felt that the "pro-HRT bandwagon was perilously out of control."[7]

That sounds like, and feels like, a devious ulterior motive to me!

In 2006, in another update of the same cohort of women, the WHI reported that they found no increased risk of breast cancer among the same women randomized to combined estrogen-progestin treatment. The alleged increased risk— "the one worth stopping the study for" had completely vanished. This news *did not* make headlines! Tara Parker-Pope noted in her 2007 book *The Hormone Decision* that the WHI "seemed to have a different standard for bad hormone news than it did for good hormone news."[8]

In 2014, Samuel Shapiro, then in the department of public health and family medicine at the University of Cape Town Medical School, and his colleagues conducted an in-depth statistical analysis of the WHI and concluded that:

> "…the over-interpretation and misrepresentation of
> the findings in the WHI study has resulted in major

damage to the health and well-being of menopausal women. The WHI was not a victory for women and their health …"

In March 2017, Robert Langer, associate dean for clinical and translational research at the University of Nevada, published an insider's view. He wrote:

"Highly unusual circumstances prevailed when the WHI trial was stopped prematurely in July 2002. The investigators most capable of correcting the crucial misinterpretations of the data were *actively* excluded from the writing and dissemination activities."[9]

Tragically, the biggest fall out of the WHI study is that women have suffered needlessly for years! Western physicians and nurses were immediately taught that you cannot prescribe hormones to women because they will kill them. Nancy Belcher, PhD. MPH states in her April 2023 article:

"These findings continue to be echoed over and over on the internet even though they are inaccurate, outdated, and were reversed by the very researchers that released the findings."

"…In my opinion, the most detrimental impact of the WHI study was the inaccurate identification of a relationship between the use of estrogen therapy and the risk for heart disease, and breast cancer."

Physicians and the media taught women that hormones are bad. More importantly, we have studies that clearly show that *bi-oidentical* hormones can give you years of vitality and can improve cardiovascular health, bone health, mood, wellness, and reduce cancer and mortality in the range of 30 to 50 percent.[10,11,12]

In my opinion, the WHI study further reinforces, as Robert Lustig calls it, the "diabolical" nature of Big Medicine and Big Pharma! My question is, if this was a study designed to look at preventative health for men, would we have seen the same egregious behaviors and outcomes?

Personally, the WHI study reinforces why we need to be our own advocates and carefully sift through what we hear from our conventional medical providers. We need to understand our bodies, listen to our bodies, and do what we can to prevent disease.

## The Gift of Functional Medicine

Only five to ten percent of chronic disease is a result of bad genes.[13] The rest is dictated by your diet and lifestyle, including your thoughts, relationships, and even your environment. Neither my graduate nor post-graduate studies taught me anything about the field of psychoneuroimmunology, yet I will educate you on this exciting field as well as the powerful impact of Epigenetics in the pages ahead.

The disease model of conventional medicine, which I now call "dysfunctional" medicine, focuses on the symptom and prescribes a treatment or prescription to alleviate the symptom. Functional medicine, on the other hand, gets to the root cause of disease. Our entire being—Spiritual, Emotional, Mental and Physical—work together to contribute to our level of overall vitality. If you're depleted in any one area, it affects your capacity for health and vitality. Therefore, Functional Medicine providers search for *underlying causes*, including addressing adverse childhood events, stress, trauma, environmental toxins, nutritional deficiencies, imbalances, etc.

In Dr. Lustig's Metabolical book, he describes the root of our dysfunctional healthcare or "sickness system" that results in such poor outcomes for mortality and morbidity—and that is, Western medicine treats the symptom, not the root cause. The symptom can be treated with a drug, a surgical procedure, or an extensive treatment plan that often only reduces symptoms, yet does not heal, or can even make matters worse.

Unfortunately, our Western-trained medical students only have 19.6 contact hours of nutrition instruction, which equals 0.27 percent of their time spent in class. Compare that with a Doctor of Chiropractic, where nutrition classes are intermingled throughout the entire curriculum to receive their license. Dr. Lustig continues to describe in detail the conflict of interest that goes on between Big Pharma, Big Food, and Big Medicine. Read Lustig's book, and your jaw might just drop. Or you might choose to start making simple changes, like what you eat.

What we do to our health today will impact us ten, twenty, and thirty years down the road! Do you want to have vitality and freedom to do what you want with your body? Do you want to be able to work; play with your kids and grandkids; to travel and enjoy better levels of freedom? Then get started today!

## *Consider This*

- Have you experienced medical visits or been prescribed medicines that don't feel quite right, in your gut?

- Are there any medications, such as birth control pills or synthetic hormones, that you'd like to eliminate?

*Three*

# Hallmarks of Vitality

*"The higher your energy level, the more efficient your body, the better you feel, and the more you will use your talent to produce outstanding results."*
~Tony Robbins

It is not uncommon to see exercise fanatics or healthy professional athletes or college-age young men drop dead suddenly. Some of you may remember Jim Fixx, the bestselling author of *The Complete Guide to Running*. He is often credited with helping start America's fitness revolution in the late seventies. Ironically and sadly, he died of a heart attack at age 52 while running. Or perhaps you remember Darryl Kile, renowned starting pitcher for the Houston Astros, who died suddenly of a heart attack at age 33 during regular season. Sergio Grinkov, two-time Olympic Gold Medalist in paired figure skating, died suddenly of a heart attack at age 28. He left behind his skating partner and wife, age 24, and a three-year-old daughter. It can be shocking to see someone who is known for their impeccable fitness level or impeccable diet being diagnosed with a devastating disease, or who suddenly passes away.

Whatever your picture of health is for you, one thing is certain—it involves more than one or two things, like running or going on a diet. While nutrition and movement are critical to optimal health, there's a bigger picture, perhaps at a DNA level.

And that bigger picture involves determining what's really going on beneath the surface, so tragedies like the ones above don't happen to you or someone you love.

Our entire being—Spiritual, Emotional, Mental, and Physical—works together to contribute to our level of overall vitality. If you're depleted in any one area, it affects your entire capacity for optimal health and vitality. You deserve nothing less than whole health.

## What Does Vitality Look Like?

The dictionary defines vitality as physical strength or vigor, and its synonyms include having sparkle, stamina, vim, and aliveness. People who experience vitality find they have the capacity to live a life of passion and purpose. It includes having a precious vital life force that sustains us and allows us to contribute to others.

It's impossible to achieve vitality when we are not experiencing optimal health. Check in on how you feel right now, compared with this list showing what vitality looks like:

- Energy available throughout the day
- Looking younger than your age
- Falling asleep quickly, and sleeping throughout the night
- Awakening refreshed
- Enjoying a wide variety of activities
- Emotional stability
- Meeting challenges without feeling anxiety or overwhelm
- A mind that is clear and alert
- A healthy glow to skin, eyes, and hair
- Balanced sexual energy
- Joy, laughter, and fun

- Meaningful, supportive, fulfilling relationships
- A strong sense of purpose
- A feeling of gratitude
- Comfortably digesting your food
- Bowel movements that are regular—
  two to three times a day
- Urination that occurs every 2-3 hours

If you experience any of these hallmarks of vitality, congratulations! This book can help you achieve even greater vitality.

If this list seems like something from an unattainable ideal, don't panic. This book provides a wonderful opportunity to learn how to dramatically increase your health and level of vitality. In fact, it's never too late or too early to use the benefits of compounding interest in what I call your "Physical Portfolio" by making one small change, or one percent improvement, in your health *every* day.

# Compound Interest

Compound interest is the 8th wonder of the world.
He who understands it, earns it; he who doesn't, pays it.
*~Albert Einstein*

Many of us have been taught about the amazing effect of compounding interest when it comes to our financial or fiscal portfolio. But have you ever thought about this principle as it relates to your physical health and vitality?

## How is your physical portfolio?

As a nurse practitioner and clinical nurse specialist, I've worked for years in the crisis management end of healthcare. Repetitive "roto-rooter" procedures (such as heart catheters and stents), multiple bypass surgeries, and even heart transplants were the norm. In the beginning, it was fun and exciting to practice in this fast-paced, high-tech specialty. But after years of seeing the same patients come back again and again, I knew we were not getting to the root of the problem. In other words, it seemed these patients were still paying very high interest rates for their poor health, and they just could not get out of physical debt.

The rules of compounding interest were at play here, but not in a good way. Years of poor choices were compounding in a negative way in my patients' bodies: things like refined, fatty, and sugary foods void of nutrition; long, stress-filled workdays; sedentary lifestyles; sleep deprivation; toxic exposures creating inflammation; and on and on and on.

Now, as an Integrative Health Coach specializing in functional medicine, I typically see clients who are in "debt" physically but want help in turning it around. Many are overweight and have the poor health habits described above. To make matters worse, many are usually on a few prescription medications that are wreaking havoc with negative side effects. This is *not* vitality!

Vitality requires that you take the time, year after year, to carefully analyze your *physical portfolio*. You may spend years working for money for retirement, only to spend your retirement years feeling debilitated, tired, out of shape, or battling a life-threatening disease.

A friend told me a story of one of his very successful colleagues who had a fabulous retirement party where he was celebrated with honors—but he never made it home from his party. He suffered a fatal heart attack while standing next to his car as he was about to drive home. Have you heard of similar tragic stories?

Our natural instincts and generations of programming make it very easy for us to put off taking care of our bodies. In an evolutionary sense, men have long been conditioned to protect and provide for their tribe. Men's brains have higher levels of testosterone, which can fuel their levels of competitiveness and protectiveness and lead them to ignore what their body is telling them. Imagine if one of our ancestors was chasing the proverbial beast to feed his family, but quit because he tripped and fell. His tribe would've starved. As discussed previously, men typically will put their physical needs on the back burner until their symptoms are screaming at them. Today, women are much the same way. We must work deliberately to override our basic human instincts to think about and address our long-term health.

Women's brains have higher levels of estrogen than men's brains, which helps women to pay careful attention to their bodies when they are focused on creating offspring. However, they too will completely shut off the alarms their body is sending while they nurture their children. Until symptoms are screaming at them, women will sacrifice their own health for those around them. While I did not have young children I was caring for, I was indeed investing all of my energy into my patients at work. Only when we can see that caring for our own health is really helping our families, our careers, and our own future selves will we take the time to care for our bodies and ourselves.

Taking care of yourself requires new habits. You get to choose every day, day after day, what you will eat and drink, if you will move your body or not, if you will abuse substances or not, and if you manage your stress or not. The choice to be your healthiest is truly yours to make.

Even if you are already in physical debt or even bankruptcy (i.e., cancer or cardiovascular disease), there is still help. Yes, it may be a long hard road to turn your health around, but it's worth it! Get the support you need to find the root cause of your health problems so that you can make vitality *your* reality. There are many basics you can do to improve the function of your genes, which will then improve or diminish symptoms across the board.

It is *fiscally* responsible to take care of your *physical* health. There really is no greater wealth than health!

## How Do You Get There?

When you feel like you're doing what seems "normal" to get or stay healthy, but you just plum do *not* feel good, it's time to figure out what's really going on. Perhaps you feel wired, tired, grumpy, exhausted all the time, and certainly nothing like giddy or happy or healthy.

You know in your gut that something is just not right. You know that you are not feeling like your younger self, yet all of your labs are "within normal limits." You might even go from doctor to doctor to be told—just like my clients and I were—that "there's nothing wrong." Perhaps you too have been given "a pill for your ill" only to feel worse from the side effects of that pill.

I know the frustration is intense. The hopelessness can be overwhelming when you've spent months, even years, bouncing from doctor to doctor trying to get answers. If you are like me, you may have even spent a lot of money to try and heal, yet still left with no clear-cut solution. You want someone who listens. You need someone's help to get to the bottom of your suffering and receive some relief. You know there's got to be a better way.

And you're right. A better way can be found with practitioners who are trained to get to the root cause.

# Consider This

- What signs or symptoms are you feeling in your own body right now that, if left uncared for, could get worse with time?

- Do you manage stress with bad habits to escape (such as screentime or processed food or a nightly glass or two of wine)?

- What habits could you change that will help you feel good?

- Picture yourself five or ten years from now, with the effect of those bad habits etched in your body, mind, and spirit. How do you feel?

- What is your picture of vitality?

# Section 2

# Epigenetic Mastery:
# Discover Your Path to Vitality

## *Four*

# Getting to the Root Cause

*"Functional medicine is often described as 21st-century medicine.
It is a science-based approach that looks at the function of
the body's systems and how they interact with one another
rather than naming a disease and giving a pill."*

~AMY MYERS, MD

I look at medicine like a tree. At the top of the tree are the branches. These branches represent conventional medicine where the "-ologists" practice. Instead of being seen as a whole tree—with roots, trunk, branches, leaves that are all expressed together (much like your whole spiritual, emotional, mental, and physical being)—it is medicine divided by the parts, often without one part or "-ologist" talking to the other. I practiced in this area of medicine for years, too, until I saw the light. Until I saw the whole tree.

Now, if you are lucky, you may find a doctor who sees things from the level of the trunk looking for core imbalances and dysfunctions. They may look at nutritional deficiencies, hormonal imbalances, detoxification issues, immune challenges, or neurotransmitters. Your care from this provider gives you a much greater chance to heal.

Optimally, you want to find someone who goes all the way to the root cause, like the roots of the tree. Examples of root causes are genetic predispositions, environmental toxins, stress, allergies, attitudes, psychological stress, emotional trauma, and adverse childhood events.

## It's Not "All In Your Head"

In helping women understand what ails them, I start by acknowledging their symptoms and letting them know they're not crazy. Just because one particular provider hasn't found the answer doesn't mean that you are crazy or that your health issue doesn't exist. It doesn't necessarily mean there isn't something off in your body, and it also doesn't necessarily mean there is something off in your mind or spirit, either. Whatever you are feeling today, don't settle for inaccurate conclusions or inadequate treatments that aren't helping you feel better. It's critical to be validated, receive empathy, and get targeted approaches to search for the root cause.

## Know There's Another Approach

A friend started getting severe headaches in late 2019 that were always on the right side of her head. They were minor at first, but after several months the headaches became worse and more frequent. When she finally saw a doctor, she was diagnosed with "cluster headaches" and given two prescriptions which did nothing to alleviate her pain. In fact, her headaches soon became debilitating and impacted her ability to live a "normal" life, given that she experienced six to eight painful episodes a day that lasted for up to 45 minutes and hurt her right-side face, brow, jaw, ear, neck, and shoulder. It wasn't until 2023 when an "old school" chiropractor asked, "Have we x-rayed your neck?" No. Another chiropractor examined her and said that the problem was in her neck, not in her brain (as fears were mounting of a potential tumor or other disease). Once the X-rays were taken, and the root cause of her headaches was discovered, she was prescribed different modalities of holistic care. Finally, after six years of chronic pain, she is achieving dramatic relief, and her neck is being healed.

Unlike the Traditional Medicine approach where several doctors attempted to treat my friend's symptoms by immediately trying to subdue or control her pain with drugs, a Functional Medicine approach looks for the source of the symptom and works by understanding the interconnected mechanisms of your body as a whole. The point is to diagnose what is disrupting your body's regular mechanisms and try to remove it from your body. Functional medicine means using treatments that focus on optimal functioning of the body and its organs—or getting to the *root cause* of disease—versus treating symptoms with a pill for an ill.

## Determine the root cause

Significant questions and targeted testing go into discovering the root cause behind your physical issues. When I worked as a nurse practitioner, we were taught to follow an algorithm. Depending on your answers to A, B, or C, the algorithm dictated our next question. If you answer yes to question A, then we follow the algorithm in that direction. If it's a no, then we may proceed down the B or C pathway, depending on your answers. We follow the algorithm using the *subjective* data (the symptoms you share and questions you answer) and combine it with *objective* data (the physical exam as well as various lab and diagnostic tests). The goal was to "rule things out" until you could narrow, narrow, narrow, and then pinpoint, zero in, and proclaim, "That's it," because everything else has been ruled out.

What's so frustrating for many women is that their doctors are not really listening. First, they only have 15 minutes to see you. If they don't have the time or instinct to listen carefully and really dig deeper, they can miss very important subjective and objective data! Women are thus left feeling that their symptoms are negated and blown off. If the symptoms don't match up with what's in the textbook, doctors will dismiss it. Or worse, as I discussed earlier, they could say what my former colleague said to me, when he said, "How many hours do you spend a day researching your illness online?" and then patted my knee and said, "You just leave your healthcare up to me."

## Go upstream

Now, as an integrative health coach, I do advanced testing. I do the DUTCH hormone test. I do DNA testing. I do the PULS cardiac test. I do heavy metal testing. I do mold testing. I also check neurotransmitters and gut microbiome levels. I dig in and find out what hasn't been tested and what else is going on with my client.

Any one or all these things I test for can shut down your cellular energy (the mitochondria). Here's a simple analogy—if the reception on your cell phone is down to one bar, or if the battery is low and needs recharging every few hours, something's wrong on a "cellular" level.

It's the same with your cells in your body. We need to figure out what's going on upstream, or the root cause, because most diagnoses that women are receiving do not address this. In my opinion, they don't have 'chronic fatigue' or some other superficial diagnosis. Instead, they've got something else that's causing the mitochondrial dysfunction at the cellular level.

Note: The toxins above cause the mitochondrial dysfunction. The fatigue and mitochondrial dysfunction are the *symptoms* of the problem. The actual problem, or diagnosis, is the inability to detox!

Even cancer, in my opinion, is just a *symptom* of a different problem. The diagnosis is actually that you may be overloaded with toxins, have poor detoxification, or lack proper nourishment. Toxins may be in the form of EMFs or bad air or heavy metals or mold or a toxic sugar-laden inflammatory diet. As a result, your immune system is in the tank, and you cannot naturally fight off the cancer stem cells that form on a regular basis.

Stress is another major contributor to chronic illness that I will discuss in detail in Chapter 16. In this fast-paced modern world we live in, it's not just medical providers who are not listening. Most of us are not listening to our own bodies! I did this, too. Remember, I ignored the messages until I was *forced* to slow down.

## Slow down

Years ago, I listened to a talk given by Dieter F. Uchtdorf, a retired airline captain who said that when the "pitch, yaw, and roll" of turbulence comes, inexperienced pilots will try and speed up. Uchtdorf said, "Professional pilots understand that there is an optimum turbulence penetration speed that will minimize the negative effects of turbulence. And most of the time that would mean to reduce your speed."[1]

The same is true for taking care of our bodies. When you are stressed, your cortisol rises. It can be from deadlines, personal issues, lack of sleep, overwhelm, etc. That's turbulence. To protect our bodies, just like an airplane, we need to slow down. Part of slowing down is listening to your body; noticing your body; noticing that you are not feeling good. If you are not feeling good, there's a high probability that your DNA is not expressing itself optimally. This book illustrates the core essential things that either sabotage or support your DNA. By understanding the core essentials, you can *own* your power and take back your health.

# Choose Your Health Instead of Your Dis-Ease

I once had a client say with a little humor in her voice, "You're so mean" when I suggested a dietary change that would optimize her health and help her heal a diagnosis of Fatty Liver Disease.

I didn't react to her upset, but I did think afterward about what she said. I was reminded of a great scripture. "There is a law irrevocably decreed in heaven before the foundations of this world, upon which all blessings are predicated—and when we obtain any blessing from God, it is by obedience to the law upon which it is predicated."[2]

When it comes to optimizing our health and our DNA expression, these are not *my* rules, these are *God's* laws. I did not make up the laws that govern the body's healthy physiology or pathophysiology (i.e., disease process). I can only illuminate these laws for you. Then you get to choose!

As Mark Hyman, MD, so eloquently puts it:

> "Most of us witness abnormal aging and we think it's normal, but it's not—it's abnormal aging. The decline in decrepitude, disability, dysfunction, and losing your health is not an inevitable part of aging. Six out of 10 Americans have a chronic illness, most people suffer from some sort of chronic illness as they get older—it's because of how we're living, our diet, environmental toxins, lack of exercise, stress, and a host of other factors that are really causing a decline in our health and we don't really see vibrant aging. We don't inevitably have to succumb to what we think of as this aging process. We can do so much to keep ourselves vital, strong, and healthy as we get older."

My guess is that, if you are reading this book, you'd like to increase your vitality and even ensure that your health span matches your lifespan! When you understand what the underlying causal factors are, then *you* get to choose and create a new future. You get to Create the Vitality You Crave.

# Consider This

- Are you experiencing any symptoms that are unaddressed?

- Are there medications you are taking that aren't working?

- Do you feel dismissed by your doctor for an ongoing issue?

- Where can you "slow down"?

*Five*

# Make the Most of Your Epigenetic Power

*"The way you think, the way you behave, the way you eat,*
*can influence your life by 30-50 years."*
~DEEPAK CHOPRA. M.D.

Experts have shown that our DNA can be dramatically affected by the lifestyle choices we make, the thoughts we choose, the words we speak, the music we listen to (really), the environment we live in, the emotions we feel, and by the self-loving things we do to heal ourselves. We have so much more control over our DNA expression than we imagine by using the science of Epigenetics.

## Understanding Epigenetics

What is Epigenetics? "EPI" is a prefix that means "upon," "over," "at," or "before." "Genetics" is the "science of heredity." Thus, Epigenetics is "the study of the way in which the expression of heritable traits is modified by environmental influences or other mechanisms without a change to the DNA sequence." More simply put, Epigenetics is "control above genetics."

I'm a musician, so I love to use the analogy of a grand piano when I explain Epigenetics.

Imagine a beautiful grand piano with the lid up all the way sitting on a stage ready for a performance. You have no idea what is going to come out of the piano or how the piano will "express" itself. It's sitting there with a beautiful frame, a bunch of wires, a keyboard, and foot pedals. The wiring, like our DNA, does not dictate the music that is expressed, whether it's Bach or Billy Joel, Beethoven or Beyoncé. For music to be expressed, it requires the external influence of the pianist. If the pianist strikes a key and it's flat, that reminds me of a gene which is not functioning up to par or is functioning slower than what is optimal. If a note is sharp, it's like a gene that is functioning a bit too fast. Occasionally, individuals have missing genes. The official term is NULL, which in essence means nada—it's simply not there. On the piano, that would mean that the entire wire is missing, and the note won't play.

Years ago, I was on a stage with other music lovers, and we encircled a big black grand piano to hear a pianist perform all of the Bach piano concertos in one evening. It was spectacular! The professional piano tuner had to be there all evening and work to tune the piano after every number. It was that important to optimize the quality of the sound.

*"Epigenetics is the study of how environmental factors talk to your DNA and change which genes are active, thereby shifting how your cells conduct the chemistry of life."*

~TERRY WHALS, MD

Our bodies were designed by God to be an even finer instrument than a Steinway & Sons Fibonacci (valued at $2.4 million). We get to choose to be like the piano tuner and unlock the expression of our healing powers by optimizing our DNA.

Bruce Lipton, PhD, an American stem cell biologist and author of *The Biology of Belief,* is known as the "Godfather of Epigenetics." In a live presentation in 2019,[1] Lipton said: "The chemistry of the blood determines the expression of your genes." Think about that for a minute. How can we change the chemistry of our blood? Part of the answer is that what we eat or drink dramatically alters the chemistry of our blood.

Dr. Bruce Lipton taught medical school biology for almost 40 years. Using a petri dish, he demonstrated that if you subject a cell to one type of agar (the growth medium), then it will behave one way. If you subject a cell to a different agar, then it will behave in a different way. If you subject your cells to a bunch of sugar or highly acidic trans fats, your cells will respond (and so will your DNA eventually) negatively. If instead you subject your cells to healthy organic green veggies, then guess what—your cells thrive!

Dr. Lipton said we are "skin covered petri dishes." So, what's in your petri dish? What are you subjecting your cells to? Intuitively we all know that an organic green drink is better than a sugar- or aspartame-laced soda, but thinking that our diet can change the expression of our genes might seem a little far-fetched. But the science shows that yes, diet has a *huge* role in the expression of our genes.

## Understand Your Genetic Blueprint

You can get a DNA test to determine your specific bio-individualized blueprint. Your genetic blueprint can help you understand where you may need to pay more attention to your diet and lifestyle factors to improve your health. Knowing your heritage is great, but having clarity on exactly what genes have mutations and how you can work around them or support them with diet, lifestyle, detoxification, and supplementation can transform your health and vitality. Even without a test, you can get a *hint* of what your health risks might be. Regardless, it's important to remember that only five percent of disease is caused by "lousy" DNA; it's what we *do* with our DNA that impacts our risk of disease.

In my case, I've known since I was a young teen that I had a whopping family history of cardiovascular disease, which impacted my dietary choices in my teens, my twenties, my thirties, and beyond. I knew my mother died of liver disease at the age of 25. As a family, we had a few suspicions of what might have "caused" it, but we had no idea of what DNA variations might have been at the root cause. No one knew because no one thought to ask.

My paternal grandmother had Alzheimer's disease, my paternal grandfather had a stroke, my maternal grandmother had diabetes and ovarian cancer, and my maternal grandfather had an aortic aneurysm. My father died of a massive heart attack at 61. My aunt, my sister, and my cousin had or are living with breast cancer. Just from looking at my family's "health" history, it's easy to say that I'm at higher risk for breast cancer, Alzheimer's disease, and cardiovascular disease.

I was naturally concerned about all of these. While it's my family medical history, I refused to accept that it was my DNA *destiny!* When I finally did a DNA test and had that bio-individualized information that revealed the genetic common denominators, I was able to find the missing puzzle pieces of *my* health picture. That has proven to be invaluable, even liberating! And it can be that way for you.

## Your DNA is Not Your Destiny

You do *not* have to be victim to your genetic blueprint. Just because your grandparents or parents have had a specific health challenge does not mean you have to expect the same health challenges. My mother died six days after I turned two years old. But I've since used that as a catalyst to turn my health around, once I understood my DNA and the principle of Epigenetics.

I'll give you more details about my genetic transformation in the pages ahead, but for now, here's another amazing statement from Dr. Lipton:

> "Your thoughts are converted into chemistry
> that control your biology."[2]

This means that using the power of our thoughts is another element we can use to change our genetic expression. Additionally, focusing on lifestyle, movement, mindfulness, relationships, and surrounding environmental toxins plays a huge role in our DNA expression. If you are living in a mold-infested environment or working in a toxic environment (the air or the other people), then this too will have a direct impact on the expression of your DNA. We will discuss what some of these "epigenetic-induced alterations" are throughout this chapter.

Margaret Smith, PhD, geneticist from Australia, wrote in her book titled *Gene Genius*:

> "All the latest findings about genes, the ability to
> influence them and, sometimes to repair damage
> to them, constitute clear irrefutable scientific
> proof that HOW we live, HOW we deal with our
> experiences, WHAT we believe and the LIFESTYLE
> WE CHOOSE can have a real and lasting impact on
> our genetic make-up. NO longer are we the passive
> recipients of the destiny it might well have once
> mapped out for us, and hard wired into us. Instead,
> we can have significant input into how healthy our
> genes will end up being."[3] (CAPS not added)

Renowned American Genetic Expert Ben Lynch, ND, sums it all up by saying:

"Your Genes are NOT your destiny!"[4]

In fact, only five percent of cancer and cardiovascular disease patients can attribute their disease solely to heredity.[5] Even the incredible media frenzy about BRCA1 and BRCA2 genes that made big news with Angeline Jolie's bilateral mastectomy failed to mention that 95 percent of breast cancers are *not* due to inherited genes. "Cancers are derived from environmentally induced epigenetic alterations, and not defective genes."[6]

Dr. Bruce Lipton further emphasizes that, "The diseases that are today's scourges—diabetes, heart disease and cancer . . . are not the effect of a single gene, but of complex interactions among multiple genes and environmental factors."[7]

So, there you have it—four experts clearly teaching us that we have the power to impact the expression of our genes.

In the meantime,

"Never affirm or repeat about your health
what you do not wish to be true."
~Ralph Waldo Trine

# Understanding DNA Test Results

In the world of DNA testing, you will hear of SNPs. SNP stands for "Single Nucleotide Polymorphism."

### What are single nucleotide polymorphisms (SNPs)?

Single nucleotide polymorphisms (pronounced "snips") are the most common type of genetic variation among people. Each SNP represents a difference in a single DNA building block, called a nucleotide. For example, a SNP may replace the nucleotide cytosine (C) with the nucleotide thymine (T) in a certain stretch of DNA.

SNPs occur normally throughout a person's DNA. On average, they occur almost once in every 1,000 nucleotides, which means there are roughly four to five million SNPs in a person's genome. These variations occur in many individuals. To be classified as a SNP, a variant is found in at least one percent of the population. Scientists have found more than 600 million SNPs in populations around the world.

Most SNPs have no effect on health or development.[8] Some of these genetic differences, however, have proven to be very important in the study of human health. SNPs help predict an individual's response to certain drugs, susceptibility to environmental factors such as toxins, and the risk of developing diseases. SNPs can also be used to track the inheritance[9] of disease-associated genetic variants within families. Research is ongoing to identify SNPs associated with complex diseases such as heart disease, diabetes, and cancer.

Before I go on, I want to clarify that the focus in this book is not to discuss various SNPs or DNA pathways, or how to support various mutations—I have a list of my favorite books at the back of the book that can do just that. My focus is to help you understand that you indeed *do* have power to improve your DNA expression. If you implement the dietary and lifestyle recommendations that I outline in this book, *each* gene expressed will be more optimized.

## To Your Future-Self

Creating your Future-Self using your epigenetic power is where the rubber meets the road. You are creating daily, whether you realize it or not. You can use your power on each level—spiritual, mental, emotional, and physical. We *can* choose to actually act upon our physical reality each and every day.

So, how do you create new habits and new patterns that will support your DNA expression rather than sabotage it? The pages ahead show the way.

> "We are free to act for ourselves and not to be acted upon."[10]

## Consider This

- What are some of the things you already know that might be impacting your risk of inheriting that certain family history disease?

- What genetic risk factors are you most concerned about altering?

- Do you know what ways you are impacting your genetic expression—positively or negatively?

# Section 3

## Nurture Your Vitality Through Creation Principles

# Six

# Use the Power of Creation Principles

*"Watch your thoughts, they become your words;*
*watch your words, they become your actions;*
*watch your actions, they become your habits;*
*watch your habits, they become your character;*
*watch your character, it becomes your destiny!"*

~Lao Tzu

Years ago, I was enthralled with the process of visualization that I learned from the master teacher Napoleon Hill in his landmark book *Think and Grow Rich*. I remember writing out a very specific visualization for my future, using all five senses with incredible specificity. I would recite this and feel inspired. My visualization did not come to fruition as easily as I had expected, and so eventually I let this practice slip.

When I was introduced to the "Power of Creation Principles," my heart was elated, because then I had a new level of tools to *create* in my daily life with consistency. For me, the Creation Principles were the missing pieces to my visualization practice. Creation Principles can be applied to your health as well as every area of your life. After all, we are *whole* beings. As you know, I believe that in order to have optimal vitality, we must address our whole being—spiritually, mentally, emotionally, and physically.

If you know the Creation Story in the Holy Scriptures, it clearly shows that God used both spiritual and physical Creation Principles. The spiritual creation uses "see, say, and feel." He visualizes what He wants to create—the world, then light, then firmament separating the water from the land, and then plants, animals, and humans—all brought about in stages. "One step at a time," "line-upon-line," "here a little, there a little," day after day. God then used physical creation, the "do," to create each of the parts of our world kingdom.

> And I, God, said: Let there be light; and there was light.
> And I, God, saw the light; and that light was good.
> And I, God, divided the light from the darkness.[1]

Personally, I've struggled with this principle, and I've also seen my clients struggle with it year after year. Have you ever made a New Year's resolution and not seen it to fruition? Most often, it's because we have not used *both* spiritual and physical creation! Going to the gym or buying healthier foods are all parts of DOing something new, but without the spiritual creation, the physical fades way too fast.

Consider an iceberg. Most of the iceberg is under the water line. Under the water line is like the spiritual creation. We must have the clarity of *see, say, and feel* before we begin the *do*. We must change what is under the surface to begin to see real changes above the surface.

Remember that we are creating daily, whether we realize it or not. We can be using our creative powers to uplift, grow, change, and spiral up, or we can be using these powers to create negative and nasty thoughts, patterns, habits, and therefore downward spirals on each level—spiritual, mental, emotional, and physical.

When we combine each of these levels with *spiritual creation* it looks like this:

- Spiritual – to SEE
- Mental – to SAY, including what we say to ourselves, as well as what we THINK on a subconscious level
- Emotional – to FEEL
- Physical – to DO

The Holy Scriptures teach us that we can choose to "act or be acted upon" each and every day![2]

# The Power of Your Thoughts

As mentioned in Chapter 5, Bruce Lipton, PhD, renowned author of *The Biology of Belief* and considered the Godfather of Epigenetics, said our mind is powerful, and "its job is to take our thoughts and turn them into chemicals that will alter our cells and our organs."

Think about that!

I've seen this in action. Numerous patients, friends, and even family members, who were diagnosed with a challenging disease or received a fatal prognosis for their disease, died on the date their doctors told them they were going to die—almost with exact specificity. Wow. Were their doctors just "right" every time? Or is there something else going on?

## The placebo effect

I'm sure most of you have heard of the placebo effect. Science has shown repeatedly that the power of the mind can cause a positive effect, even if the person may be taking just a sugar pill. Big Pharma takes great effort to "control" for the placebo effect. What if medicine had spent years looking into the power of the placebo effect to actually heal the patients?

Here's a story of a shocking study into the significance of the "placebo effect" which has changed the course of medicine. In the late 1950s, surgeons were cutting or "ligating" the internal mammary arteries (on the chest wall) to provide for blood flow to the coronary muscle for patients who were suffering from angina or chest pain.[3]

Then in 1960, a small study compared angina patients who had their internal mammary arteries cut versus patients who had a small incision on their chest wall, but the artery was *not* cut. Shockingly, 71 percent of those subjected to the sham surgery got better, whereas only 67 percent of those who got the real surgery improved. Now that's the power of the placebo effect.[4]

## The nocebo effect

The nocebo effect is just as powerful, but it is the opposite of the placebo effect. If a patient is told or if they believe that a certain pill or procedure will cause irreparable harm or a negative outcome, or if they're told their disease is terminal, then their mind may begin to bring about exactly what Dr. Lipton stated— "change the biochemistry so that the body will respond to match those thoughts." Clearly, we all need to be very careful about the thoughts we let in everyday and which ones we plant and which ones we nourish.

I have seen countless patients who were expected to die, but then completely blew the medical community away with their recovery, being discharged from the ICU, healing well, and going on to live a healthy life, even when there seemed to be no hope that their body could heal.

## Your thoughts in effect

Do we have the power to make ourselves sick? It turns out we do! Dr. Bernie Siegel shared in his sentinel book, *Love, Medicine & Miracles*, a study showing that patients in a control group for a new chemotherapy drug were given nothing but saline (salt water), yet they were warned that it *could* be the actual drug. Thirty percent of them lost their hair! In another study, hospitalized patients were given sugar water and told it would make them vomit—80 percent of them vomited.[5]

Clearly these stories illustrate the power of our thoughts—whether to heal or make us sick.

In my early days in nursing, a 34-year-old patient (I'll call him Tom) who had Adult Respiratory Distress Syndrome (ARDS) was close to dying from severe pneumonia. He was in the ICU and expected to only live a few more days. We were using a pediatric ventilator to keep his respiratory rate near 100 because we could not oxygenate him on an adult ventilator. He was in a very critical state. He wrote a note to his young wife and asked if she would "let him go." As the Clinical Nurse Specialist, I was able to bend the rules a bit and bring his two daughters, ages five and seven, into the ICU to see him. We put the bed down as far as it would go, lowered the railings, and allowed the little girls to hug their dad. They put their heads on his lap. It was incredibly tender to see him caress their hair and love on these little girls. The visit was short and sweet, and then I had to escort these little girls out of the ICU, knowing that this could be the last time they would see their daddy alive. I asked his wife to bring in a picture of the family. We taped it to his ventilator pole that comes across the bed to hold up the tubing. This little family picture was now in direct view of Tom's vision. At the end of the long day, I checked in on Tom, and his breathing had not changed. He continued to decline. I went home for the day on a Friday afternoon. When I returned to work on Monday morning, Tom was not in the ICU room. I expected to hear of his passing. To my utter shock, I found out that in less than 24 hours after his family had visited and their picture was taped to where he could see it, his breathing normalized, he was able to oxygenate his body, the ventilator tubes were removed, and he was transferred out of the ICU to a regular room! *Wow, I thought. What caused this?*

In my years of critical care and since, I have seen many people who doctors had written off for death, only to spring back unexpectedly. Likewise, I've seen others who were doing well and just as suddenly took a turn for the worse and died. I have seen people, even those close to me, who were told by their medical providers that they only have "three weeks to live," and they pass exactly on the third week deadline. Coincidence?

## Epigenetics at work

We discussed the power of Epigenetics in Chapter 5. This burgeoning scientific field had not even begun in 1993 when I was the Clinical Nurse Specialist over Tom's care, but I instinctively knew that Tom had used his thoughts and his own will to heal his lungs and get out of the death bed in our ICU. Now, years later, as we've discovered, there are studies and stories to prove this.

> "The Pharmacy in your mind is a major player
> in the game of genetic expression."
> ~Brenda Stockdale

Our thoughts *can* change the expression of our DNA. So can our breathing, food, sleep, movement, and external toxins. Stay tuned for Chapter 18 to learn more about what you can *do* to Create the Vitality You Crave.

> "Within each of us is a spark. Call it a divine spark if you
> will, but it is there and can light the way to health. There
> are no incurable diseases, only incurable people."
> ~Bernie Siegel, M.D.

# Visualizing Your Future-Self

Do you have trouble visualizing what your future could be? Some of us might see pictures in living color and even 3D. Some of us might see words instead. Whenever we set a new goal, many of us struggle to achieve it or even see it because the goal is too far out on the timeline. It seems unrealistic. Our current self may not be able to see all of what our Future-Self envisions. But we can use either pictures or words to help visualize and create our Future-Self.

> *"Words are the Oxygen of Creation."*
>
> ~Katie Richardson

## Using the Creation Principles

Now that you know the power of using your own thoughts, you can use the Creation Principles to create your Future-Self and optimize your vitality:

- **SEE** – What is one area of your life you would most like to cultivate and grow right now?
- **SAY** – Describe your Future-Self using present tense language ("I am…")
- **FEEL** – What does your Future-Self believe and feel? Use present tense language. ("I am…")
- **DO** –What are the daily habits or behaviors that your Future-Self does every day to create the outcomes and growth? Use present tense language. ("I am…")
- **BECOME** – Who do you really want to become in your life? What do you visualize yourself being able to do? What character traits do you want to own? What habits or skills do you want to master?

I know at first it might seem like too much work, but I do promise that using these Creation Principles will have a high return on your investment. I have found that when I am really clear about who my Future-Self is, and I've taken the time to write down the specifics—using the five senses and the four bodies (Spiritual, Emotional, Mental, and Physical)—then I can read this every morning as I start my day. I can mediate on my Future-Self and have it anchor my day and my choices. At the end of the day, I can meditate again to review my actions and see the gains I made or even do a mental "do over" to strengthen me in my creative powers for the next day.

Now that you have a basic understanding of the Creation Principles, it's time to learn how to put them into use. In the next chapter, I will share tips to create consistent healthy habits, without perfectionism!

## Consider This

- Who do you want your Future-Self to be?

- What thoughts are you now noticing that might be creating negative results in your life?

- What thoughts are you going to plant and nourish each day to create the vitality you crave?

- Can you begin to visualize the actions that will support your Future-Self vision?

*Seven*

# Creator Habits that Work

*"Your whole life is a manifestation of the
thoughts that go on in your head."*

~LISA NICHOLS

I have experienced first-hand, both personally and with my clients, the profound impact of creator habits. Not only do they help transform self-sabotaging habits, but they also create a magnificent space to develop healthy patterns. We'll examine my favorite creator habits in this chapter. But before we do, let's take a look at some unhealthy creation patterns and habits.

## Unhealthy Creation Patterns and Habits

Are you being a conscious creator and being responsible for your actions, or are you consciously or unconsciously repeating old patterns that are self-sabotaging and keeping you stuck?

- **Spiritually**
  - Are you neglecting your spiritual self, such as neglecting meditation, nature, prayer, or communion with God?
  - Are you neglecting the quiet, restorative alone time that you may need to fill your cup?
- **Emotionally**
  - Are you reacting, versus responding, to the negative baiting from others?
  - Are you easily taking offense?

- **Mentally**
  - Are you using negative self-talk?
  - Are you assuming the worst in any given situation?
- **Physically**
  - Are you eating sugar-laden and processed foods?
  - Are you skipping meals altogether or doing late-night bingeing of unhealthy snacks?
  - Are you going to bed after midnight and getting only five to six hours of sleep or less?
  - Are you drinking a lot of sodas or alcohol instead of clean, filtered water?

My family history includes abdominal fat, diabetes, heart disease, and cancer. I have been able to keep my weight under control with diet and exercise, but I was tracking my blood sugar every six months and watched as it gradually crept up. I rarely, if ever, eat sugar. So, I couldn't figure the cause of my increasing blood sugar levels. Then, I started tracking my food.

I examined the prepared food I was eating, for example—Nut Thins. Though gluten-free, these crunchy little crispy yummies that come in nice shiny packages are very processed and high carb. If I had eaten plain nuts, I would have been fine. But the processing of the nuts with the added rice flour was the problem, raising my blood sugar. Years ago, I used to make my own hummus, but in those Nut Thin munching days, I would buy the hummus, which was also high carb and very processed.

Then I discovered the Power of Ten. I could see that, while my taste buds were happy and satisfied at 10 seconds and 10 minutes, it was the 10 hours, 10 weeks, and 10 months afterward that were the problem. I chose to give up the processed crackers and hummus and replace them for fresh pressed almond butter and celery sticks. Yummy and crunchy! Ten months later, I was way happier with how I felt and how my blood sugar had dropped. You can feel better using The Power of Ten as a new creator habit, too.

## The Power of Ten

Sometimes trying to visualize your Future-Self a few months or a few years from now can be challenging. But, if you can use the compounding **"Power of 10"**—10 seconds, 10 minutes, 10 hours, 10 days, 10 weeks—to make it a lot easier than 10 months or 10 years. Consider then, *how do you want to feel in 10 seconds? 10 minutes? 10 hours?*

I have my clients put the number 10 on their fridge, their pantry door, and even where they may don their athletic clothes to remind them to ask themselves in that moment of choice—whether to eat a particular food, drink a beverage, avoid exercising, watch TV, or do a meditation—how do I want to feel in 10 minutes? How do I want to feel in 10 hours? How will eating this food make me feel in 10 minutes? Will it help me have greater energy in 10 hours? Will drinking this soda with caffeine and sugar affect my sleep later? How will bingeing on Netflix late at night leave me feeling? You may be enjoying yourself in 10 minutes, but what about in 10 hours? Will you feel rejuvenated the next day? Or will you be slogging around, even perhaps engaging in a bunch of negative self-talk because you chose to stay up too late or eat too much sugar?

Here's a client's story.

Erika (not her real name) was struggling with staying up way too late, either on her phone, computer, or watching TV, while mindlessly eating late-night sugary snacks at the same time. As a result, she was missing the value of deep sleep that not only comes from getting to bed before midnight, but also not sleeping soundly when she was in bed due to the toxic overload in her system. The next day, you can imagine that her mood and her productivity suffered.

She posted the number 10 on her desktop. When she was tempted to keep scrolling later in the evening, she noticed that number 10 and stopped herself. She started to go to bed earlier. Her sleep improved and so did her mood and productivity. Not only that, because her sleep improved, her desire and capacity to engage in other health habits increased, too.

# Address Triggers

## Assess negative triggers

In the world of advertising, they have mastered the art of suggesting certain habits to match triggers. Commercials seem to follow the **If** this _____ **Then** _____ scenario.

**If** you are with a group of friends enjoying a ball game and it's hot outside, **Then** you need a Coca-Cola (or some other cold drink).

Or

**If** you are at the movie theatre,

**Then** you need popcorn, soda, or candy.

These may seem fun and appetizing, but they have a significant negative effect on our DNA expression and thus our health!

Let's look at a few more:

**If** my kids are screaming,

**Then** I get anxious, upset, and yell at them to be quiet.

Or

**If** I stay up late watching TV,

**Then** when the alarm goes off, I hit snooze and skip my morning workout.

Or

**If** my kids or spouse leave a mess all over the house,

**Then** I think negative thoughts about them or bark and snark at them.

Even though these are a very common habits in our current Western culture, can you see that if you keep unconsciously doing these habits, over time they can lead to health challenges? To be specific, I mean insulin resistance, weight gain, raised cortisol and the negative cascade it causes, perhaps hypertension, cardiovascular disease, and on and on. The big take home message is this—negative triggers, left unaddressed, can have a significant effect on your DNA expression, your health, and your vitality.

## Assess positive triggers

Positive triggers can be used to help us create new *healthy* creator patterns. Previously, when I tried to create a new habit, I would set a reminder, such as an alarm on my phone. If there was a change to my schedule (planned or not), I'd simply silence the alarm or reminders, perhaps even a few times. When these reminders, that I intentionally set, interrupted my train of thought or the current result I was trying to produce, they often caused stress instead of direction. That is *not* an optimal way to create a new healthy habit. Sometimes it felt like a negative hit, times three, when I was disrupted by the alarm, when I silenced it, and then again when I faced the disappointment that I was failing at my new goal. I'm grateful that I finally learned how to create by using positive triggers.

You can use positive triggers based on:
- Timing
- Location
- Theme
- Activity

# Habit Stacking

Another great tool to create new powerful habits is "Habit Stacking," as taught by James Clear in his bestselling book *Atomic Habits*. The concept involves attaching a desired new behavior to a habit you already engage in regularly. This way, you capitalize on the reliability of your existing habits to easily integrate new ones into your daily routine.

Here's an example from my own transformation. When I first learned about the detoxification benefits of oil pulling, I was intrigued and thought it would be great to implement in my health routine. (I discuss the benefits in Chapter 8.) I struggled to do it consistently until I learned the trick of adding a positive trigger and habit stacking. Instead of having a silly alarm nagging at me that may not fit my timeline for the day, I used the positive trigger of timing instead.

*After I use my toothbrush, I will put my toothbrush away and take a tablespoon of coconut oil to do my oil pulling.*

Voila—it worked! First thing in the morning, I let my puppy out, then I brush my teeth, and then I do oil pulling for five to ten minutes while I make the bed and get dressed for my workout. I took these positive triggers and habit stacking to another level by creating supportive, vitality-enhancing rituals in my mornings and evenings.

# Meditation and Morning Rituals

As women, moms, professionals, and caretakers, we are often balancing the care of generations on either side of us and often feel that self-care is not an option. Our culture often reinforces sacrifice and service to the point of sacrificing *self*.

This I know for sure: *running on empty and a lack of self-care have left me feeling upset, unwell, and off-balance and with little access to being my best self!*

In my thirties, I had a habit of driving my body for outrageous long hours and serving others to the brink of exhaustion. I was certainly not thriving, and the principle of compound interest (as discussed in Chapter 3) meant I had to pay the price!

Male bodies were genetically designed to do that. Testosterone can fuel a man for many long hours (think of our ancestors out hunting wild game until they could finally catch it). Men have at least sixteen times the testosterone that women have. That is why they are able to produce these kinds of results and go, go, go for hours before they tax their adrenal glands. Female bodies, on the other hand, are *not* designed to do that. Women start producing the stress hormone cortisol much earlier than men. As I will share in more detail in Chapter 14 on the importance of balancing your hormones, demanding and overscheduled days with myriad deadlines can create a higher risk for hormone-related cancers. While we need daily doses of self-care to replenish and sustain ourselves, self-care is also a long-term investment for better health.

Meditation and other morning rituals are not just about feeling good in the moment. Instead, they are cumulative and have a huge compound effect on your health and vitality in all areas—Spiritually, Emotionally, Mentally, and Physically.

## Creating daily self-care rituals

Before I share my morning and evening rituals, I want to acknowledge that you may be in a different life phase than I am now as I write this book. You may be a single 45-year-old mother of two with a full-time job outside the home, or a married 35-year-old with a focus on your partnership and a burgeoning career. Setting aside time in the morning and the evening just for yourself may seem unwieldy. As a 64-year-old woman living alone in Florida, I have more time to spare in the mornings and evenings than I used to. This list of rituals is meant to inspire you with possibilities, not create guilt for what you may not be able to fit into *your* schedule.

## My morning ritual

I know that I'm not the only one who has had a harried morning that throws off an entire day. It could be a sick child who needs to stay home or a pet with soiled linens to change. Maybe your alarm didn't go off or your car won't start. When these things happen, it seems the whole day is just "off balance."

I've learned that creating some boundaries and structure around my morning has served me well beyond the time spent. In other words, the return on investment (ROI) has proven to be huge. By taking time to meditate and create my day, each day flows so much better. For instance, I keep my phone out of my bedroom and switched to airplane mode or at least in "sleep" mode. I don't turn it back on again until *after* I've started my day the way I want to. I am very conscious about what my thoughts are early in the morning. I'm conscious and very careful about the influences that I let in. Instead of responding to the influences and demands of the world, I keep the social media apps off and instead tune inward. I take the quiet time to reflect, meditate, and co-create my day with God. I nourish my body with water. I energize my body with movement. And I'm very clear about the types of messages I say to myself.

Here are some of the specifics of my morning ritual:
- Potty—me and my doggie, Gemma
- Turn on some ambient lights and battery-operated candles
- Brush my teeth

- When I put my toothbrush down, it's a trigger for me to do oil pulling with coconut oil while I make my bed
- Take my bioidentical hormones
- Apply calming essential oils
- Put on my workout clothes
- Listen to scriptures
- Prepare my nutritionals for the day
- Have 16 oz. of water with the nutritionals
- Make my green drink and leave it on the counter if I'm fasting for a few more hours
- Turn on my diffuser with therapeutic essential oils
- Read my 12-step thoughts for the day
- Review my daily affirmations and review the day I want to create
- Meditate
- Study scripture
- Walk my little Gemma, then come home and do additional movement for my body. It may look like:
  – The mini trampoline to enhance lymph flow
  – Ride the Peloton
  – Pilates
  – Weightlifting
- Then I shower and get dressed for the day

This may seem like a lot, yet I have found that the investment in my self-care has yielded so much more than I imagined. I'm calm, serene, focused, alert, and ready to co-create with God in all that I do.

## Evening and Bedtime Rituals

The best morning routines actually start with a good evening routine. There's plenty of science to show that optimal sleep begins by slowing down a bit earlier in the evening. I remember going and going up until the very last moment and then dropping into bed. Can you relate?

In our world today, we are bombarded with digital devices, endless bad news, texts and chats, Marco Polos, updates, and swipe-rights that can keep us scrolling for hours. The blue light alone wreaks havoc with melatonin and interrupts our sleep cycle, not to mention the dopamine hits and then withdrawals. Now, wearing blue-blocking glasses and turning off my devices earlier in the evening are part of my nighttime ritual.

## My nighttime ritual

I begin the following steps at least one hour before my bedtime to support my mind and body for deep sleep:

- I avoid email
- I avoid the news (I haven't watched TV since 1990)
- I turn off my social media apps so that I can relax
  and get in tune with myself and with God
- I turn down the lights with a dimmer switch
- I celebrate my activity for the day by checking my
  Oura ring. (I leave the Bluetooth off all day to avoid
  the EMF exposure. More on this in Chapter 9.)
- I brush my teeth and use the Waterpik
- I meditate for 15 minutes
- I write in my gratitude journal
- I write in my creation journal to create
  a fabulous tomorrow
- I turn the air conditioner to 68 degrees
- Put some essential oils on my body
- Then I end my day with prayer

This evening routine soothes me Spiritually, Emotionally, Mentally, and Physically and has made all the difference in the quality of my sleep.

Before you get overwhelmed and think, "oh my, I could never fit all of this into my day" or "are you nuts, I don't have that kind of luxury of time," let me share with you one of my favorite creator habit "hacks" to create consistency without perfectionism.

## Floors and Ceilings

Let's talk about New Year's resolutions again. If you are like most people, and like me in the past, I'd make a goal or resolution to start a new healthy habit at the start of the year. I'd pull it off for a while, and then BAM—life happened! Illness, overtime, family emergencies, vacation—something interrupted my perfect streak, and then the habit was thwarted because I couldn't keep up with the ideal version I created.

This is how daily gratitude journaling used to be for me. Psychoneuroimmunobiology, a relatively new field of science, is

*"In Principles Have Clarity, in Practice Have Charity."*

~CHIEKO N. OKASAKI

masterful at looking at the connection of body, mind, and spirit on our overall well-being. One such area that has been studied is that of gratitude journaling. (I'll discuss this in Chapter 16.)

I knew that gratitude journaling was beneficial, but life would happen and seem to get in the way. I could not journal consistently, until I learned about "Floors and Ceilings" from Brooke Snow, Creation Coach.

Here are the tenets of "Floors and Ceilings":

- Ceilings are the very best version of the goal, the ideal, the version that you can do "once in a while" when things seem to flow just right. A ceiling can be raised once you master your new habit at one level and want to take it up to a new level of mastery.

- Floors, on the other hand, are the rock bottom, foundation, the one-minute version that can be done when you're super busy.
- Stairs are in between floors and ceilings.
- Starter Steps are the baby steps to your floor. If you're trying to increase your movement, and your floor is walking to the mailbox and back, your starter step may be just putting your shoes on and walking around the house.

## Examples of floors, mid-steps, and ceilings

### Journaling

- My ceiling is sitting down and reviewing my day and asking some specific questions about my thoughts and actions for the day, then journaling my daily gratitude at the end.
- My floor is three simple bullet points dictated info my Day One Journaling App.
- Most days I dictate eight to twelve very detailed things that I'm grateful for. What used to be bullet points have turned into sentences and even paragraphs. On many a day I'll even start dictating things I'm grateful for in the moment. This way I can see the hand of God in my life all day, and the immediate sense of gratitude fuels my joy bucket all day.

Movement

- My ceiling is one hour of movement daily—
  that may be a combination of structured
  exercise routines combined with walking my
  little Gemma or an entire hour of pilates.
- My floor is one minute on the Mini-trampoline
- My usual is 30 to 40 minutes every day.
- Because of the floors, I'm thrilled I'm consistent,
  I know I'm making a huge impact on my health,
  and I get to celebrate the consistency!

# Practicing Your Creator Habits

Now that you understand creator habits, it's time to combine them with the Future-Self you want to become. For my own transformations and commitment to excellence and growth, I have found that when I visualize my Future-Self every day, I am committing to myself, and God, to follow through on who I say I am becoming. There are plenty of days that I need a "do-over" meditation at night, but I have found that with "floors" in place, I rarely completely skip something I'm committed to. Here's the other bonus when I am doing my self-care—I become grounded and serene and able to choose and respond, rather than react. If you need an accountability partner to help you as you create a new version of yourself, go for it. Search out the best one for you. You can connect with me as well (see the Resources section) to help you establish creator habits and make self-care a priority.

Did you know that 80 percent of people don't make it past the first chapter in a book? That means you're ready and extraordinary! I offer support in various ways to meet your specific needs, from bio-individualized private coaching to group coaching, keynote speaking, and corporate events.

While these Daily Vitals are just the beginning, they're a powerful place to start. If you're ready for more personalized support to create habits that truly support your Future-Self, see the resource section to book your free consult.

If you want more information start here: https://LoriFinlay.com/Start

## Consider This

- What are some of your If _____
  Then _____ statements that may not be very supportive or even sabotaging?

- By using the Future-Self Vision and creator habits, what are some If _____
  Then _____ habits that you can create to optimize your life?

- If you choreograph your morning ritual, what might it look like?

- What would you add to your evening routine? Aromatherapy? A luxurious bath? Candlelight? Music? Snuggling? Sex?

# Section 4

## The Power of Cleansing

*Eight*

# Cleanse Your Body

"Less pharma, more farms. Less pills, more plants.
Less GMO, more organic."

~ANONYMOUS

If you Google "cleansing" or "detoxing," you will get anywhere from 49,000 to 74,000 results, respectively. There is a trend to *do* a cleanse—whether for three days, a week, or longer—with a structured regimen of foods and supplements.

Yet, I feel that we cannot cleanse our bodies without adequate hydration flowing in and out every day. Think of a stagnant body of water. It typically looks bad, smells bed, and may even have bugs on top of it. If you believe any of the work of Dr. Matsuro Emoto[1] and his images of frozen water crystals, you can imagine that the energy of this stagnant water is very, very low and void of vitality! Do you want to feel like that? Not me. So, let's start cleansing with water.

## Drink Filtered Water

Most of us have had the experience of drinking or showering in hard chlorinated water. Many of us have also experienced the difference when drinking or showering with filtered, soft, alkaline water. The difference is night and day! With the chlorinated hard water, your hair dries out, and your skin can get itchy and scaly, if not downright painful. I know, I've lived that extreme.

Any water filter we use in our homes—whether a filter for the entire house or individual faucets and shower heads—need to be changed. Some filters require changing depending on the number of gallons used, and others may indicate a date; however, the bottom line is, when the filter gets clogged the water begins to taste or feel nasty again—even toxic.

There are fancy filters on the market that will filter chloride, Perfluorooctane Sulfonate (PFO)/Perfluorooctanoic Acid (PFOA)[2] lead, numerous heavy metals, inorganic metals, and other total dissolved solids (TDS). That's the good news—a quality filter will filter these toxins out. If you're not using a filter, you are loading your body with toxins. You will have to cleanse your system or suffer the burden of these toxins. If you have a filter and don't change it regularly, the toxins will overwhelm it, and you will absorb these toxins once again.

Bottom line, we must have good clean water, and plenty of it, to cleanse. I'll go into more depth on this later.

While I can also endorse regular cleanses packed with nutritious ingredients and healthy habits (and filtered water), there is much more to the cleansing story. But as you know by now, this book is about your entire being—spiritual, emotional, mental, and physical. I will focus on each of these elements for cleansing, yet I want to start with cleansing your body and opening up your organs and systems. That way, you can benefit most from the types of cleansing you pursue.

## Your Cleansing Organs

Have you ever done a "detox" that left you feeling even worse, instead of the promised outcome—whether it was supposed to be vitality, weight loss, or better skin, etc.? Often that is because these programs or products may help you to detox *only* on a cellular level, but they don't "open the channels" first, as they say in functional medicine. Let me explain.

Your cleansing organs are your:

- Kidneys
- Liver
- Lungs
- Skin

Each of these cleansing organs (the "channels") need to be "open" and functioning optimally so that the toxins can leave your body. If you do a cleanse and dump toxins from your cells into your blood stream, but your cleansing organs or "channels" are not "open" or functionally optimal, then you will indeed feel worse. Its medical name is a "Herxheimer" reaction or a "healing crisis" where you are left with awful symptoms of toxicity. Not good. I remember how awful I felt during one of these reactions. I had no idea what was going on. This is another reason why a bio-individualized approach is so critical when working toward restoring your vitality.

Below are some simple methods you can implement to "open the channels" of your detox organs so you can indeed release the toxic load in your body.

## Your kidneys

The kidneys play a vital role in the body's natural detoxification processes by filtering and eliminating waste products and excess fluids through urine. To support the cleansing and detoxing capacities of the kidneys, proper hydration is key. A well-hydrated body ensures that the kidneys can effectively flush out toxins and prevent the formation of kidney stones. Including kidney-friendly foods in the diet, such as berries, leafy greens, and watermelon, provides essential nutrients while contributing to overall kidney health. Limiting the intake of processed foods helps prevent undue stress on the kidneys. I drink a cup of dandelion herbal tea each morning because of the mild diuretic and cleansing effects that support kidney function. Regular exercise also promotes healthy blood circulation, benefiting the kidneys.

## Your liver

Maintaining optimal liver health is paramount for effective body cleansing, as the liver plays a central role in filtering and detoxifying harmful substances. A balanced and nutrient-rich diet, coupled with a healthy lifestyle, is crucial for supporting the liver in its intricate functions.

The liver processes nutrients, metabolizes medications, and filters toxins from the blood so they don't accumulate in the body. Poor dietary choices, such as excessive consumption of processed foods, alcohol, high-fat diets, and dairy, can burden the liver and hinder its ability to perform these vital tasks. Regular exercise and adequate hydration also contribute to liver health, promoting optimal blood flow and toxin elimination. By prioritizing a liver-friendly lifestyle, individuals can enhance the organ's innate capacity to cleanse the body, fostering overall well-being and longevity.

Personally, I do a detailed liver cleanse two times a year that includes juicing and colonics. Yet, daily regular cleansing is vital in today's toxic world.

### Improving bile flow

Bile, produced in the liver and stored in the gallbladder, helps break down fats from our food, making it easier for our bodies to absorb essential nutrients like vitamins A, D, E, and K. Improving bile flow is crucial for vitality because bile plays a key role in digestion and detoxification processes in the body. Proper bile flow also supports the elimination of toxins and waste products from the liver, promoting overall detoxification and supporting healthy liver function. Furthermore, sluggish bile flow can lead to issues like estrogen dominance and hormonal imbalances. When bile flow is compromised, the body may struggle to efficiently metabolize hormones like estrogen, leading to their accumulation in the body. This imbalance can disrupt the delicate hormonal equilibrium, potentially resulting in symptoms such as irregular menstrual cycles, mood swings, and reproductive health issues. Therefore, optimizing bile flow is not only essential for digestive health but also critical for maintaining hormonal balance and overall vitality. Additionally, toxic, synthetic foreign estrogens, called "xenoestrogens" (that we will discuss in detail in Chapter 14) can lead to sluggish bile flow, thus eliminating these toxic sources will support healthy bile flow.

---

Here's a list of ways to use your "Food as Medicine" and supplements to improve your bile flow:

- **Artichoke** – Artichokes are renowned for their digestive benefits, such as supporting liver function, gallbladder health, and bile production.
- **Beet greens** – Beet greens offer remarkable benefits for liver and gallbladder health. They can be enjoyed fresh, steamed, or sautéed. Consider incorporating beet greens into your nutritious smoothies!
- **Choline** – Choline not only stimulates bile production but also aids in improving a fatty liver. Incorporate choline-rich foods like egg yolks into your diet or opt for choline supplements.
- **Dandelion greens** – Dandelion greens, widely available, are excellent for promoting optimal liver function. Enjoy them as a salad or sauté them with other vegetables for a delicious side dish.

- **Ginger** – Ginger has the ability to directly stimulate the liver and enhance bile secretion. Enjoy ginger in teas, smoothies, or as a flavorful addition to savory sauces.
- **Lemon/Lime** – Citrus fruits like lemon and lime are simple yet effective in stimulating the liver and enhancing bile production. Add a squeeze of fresh lemon juice to your water or salad for a refreshing boost.
- **Milk thistle** – Milk thistle is a valuable supplement for liver detoxification, aiding in bile production and flow to support liver health.
- **Turmeric** – Turmeric, known for its potent phytonutrients, can alleviate liver and gallbladder inflammation while restoring healthy bile flow.

Supplements to improve bile flow:
- **Fiber** – Increasing fiber in our diet helps improve bile flow. If you are not consuming at least 25 to 30 grams a day, then increasing fiber with an organic supplement can be helpful.
- **Betaine hydrochloride** – Betaine, an amino acid found in beets, spinach, and shellfish, supports healthy digestion and stimulates bile flow.
- **Bile salts** – Bile salt supplements replenish bile in the digestive system, aiding in fat digestion. Consider incorporating bile salts into your meals. (See the Resources section.)

### How keto and intermittent fasting promote bile flow

Healthy Keto™ or Keto Green, dubbed by Anna Cabeca, M.D, diets and intermittent fasting naturally encourage the concentration and release of bile. Keto diet stimulates bile production through healthy fats, while intermittent fasting allows for intervals between meals for bile concentration. Moreover, these approaches promote a diverse microbiome and support gut health, crucial for bile acid synthesis and recycling.

### Glutathione (GSH) support

As I mentioned earlier, my mother died of Hepatitis, a liver disease, at the age of 25 years old. At the time, conventional medicine did not understand much about the role of Glutathione (pronounced Glute-a-thigh-on) for liver health and detoxification.

Because of my mother's premature death, and to ensure my own vitality and longevity, one of the most important things that I gift my body on a daily basis is a unique Glutathione support.

Glutathione (GSH) is quite a miraculous molecular super-cellular protector for *every* cell in the body. It has four major roles—master antioxidant, master detoxifier, master immune booster, and master anti-inflammatory. Glutathione (GSH) is a Tripeptide—three amino acids tied together. The amino acids Cysteine, Glutamic acid (or Glutamate), and Glycine attach to make up this miraculous molecular super-cellular protector. If your cells make enough, they thrive; if they don't, they age and die. It's that simple.

Glutathione has been considered the longevity molecule. Unfortunately, one of the reasons we see the diseases of aging increase with age is because of the drop in Glutathione. After age 20, GSH drops by about 10 percent every decade. When you're 50, you've lost approximately 40 percent of your GSH. Diet and lifestyle have a significant impact on how fast Glutathione declines.

Stress, sleep deprivation, poor diet, environmental toxins, excessive exercise, and substance abuse can all accelerate the decline. Additionally, 40 percent of Caucasians and 80 percent of Asians[3] have a genetic variant that reduces GSH function to 30 percent of normal function from the get-go. My family falls into that category, which is another reason why I enhance my Glutathione every day!

Glutathione serves as a critical component for liver health by optimizing cellular detoxification pathways, aiding in the removal of toxins, heavy metals, and other harmful substances from the body. By efficiently supporting both antioxidant defense mechanisms and detoxification processes, Glutathione helps maintain the liver's optimal functioning, ensuring overall liver health and promoting the body's detoxification capabilities.

I will share more on the importance of GSH in other chapters and include resources for obtaining the best GSH support product I have found in seventeen years of study and searching, so you can begin reducing *your* toxic load. See Resources for recommendations.

## Castor oil packs

Castor oil packs are recognized for their potential to support liver cleansing and overall detoxification. When applied topically to the skin over the liver area, typically with a cloth soaked in castor oil, these packs stimulate circulation and lymphatic drainage. The unique composition of castor oil, including ricinoleic acid, has anti-inflammatory and antioxidant properties, aiding in the reduction of inflammation and oxidative stress in the liver. The packs also promote relaxation, helping to alleviate stress, which is beneficial for liver health. Additionally, the warmth generated by the pack may enhance blood flow, encouraging the liver to efficiently process and eliminate toxins.

Regular use of castor oil packs is considered by some as a natural and gentle method to support liver function and facilitate the body's inherent cleansing processes. However, it's advisable to consult with a healthcare professional before incorporating such practices, especially for individuals with pre-existing health conditions.

I personally have used and recommend castor oil packs to my clients to support detoxification, especially if I see evidence of toxic xenoestrogens on their DUTCH hormone test. See Resources for recommendations.

## Your lungs

Deep diaphragmatic breathing is a potent method for cleansing the lungs and rejuvenating the body. By engaging the diaphragm, the primary muscle responsible for respiration, deep breathing facilitates the exchange of oxygen and carbon dioxide in the lungs, promoting efficient oxygenation of the blood. This process helps remove stale air and toxins trapped in the lungs, enhancing respiratory function and promoting overall lung health. Moreover, deep breathing stimulates the lymphatic system, aiding in the removal of waste and toxins from the body. The rhythmic expansion and contraction of the diaphragm also massage the internal organs, promoting detoxification and improving circulation. Incorporating deep diaphragmatic breathing into daily practice can help clear the lungs of impurities, boost energy levels, and support the body's natural cleansing processes, contributing to overall well-being and vitality. For more deep breathing techniques, see Chapter 18.

## Your skin

The skin, often referred to as the body's largest organ, plays a crucial role in detoxification, serving as a protective barrier against harmful external substances while also facilitating the elimination of toxins from within. Through its complex structure, comprising layers of cells and specialized glands, the skin acts as a formidable defense mechanism against environmental pollutants, microbes, and toxins. Sweat glands, particularly eccrine glands, play a significant role in detoxification by excreting waste products, such as urea, ammonia, and lactic acid, through perspiration. Additionally, sebaceous glands secrete oils that help to flush out impurities and maintain the skin's natural pH balance. The skin's intricate network of blood vessels further supports detoxification by aiding in the removal of toxins from the bloodstream through processes like diffusion and filtration. Overall, the skin's many functions make it an indispensable player in the body's detoxification processes, emphasizing the importance of proper skincare and hygiene for overall health and vitality.

## Heat therapy

Any type of heat therapy has tremendous benefits, including dry sauna, steam, hot baths, hot springs, and even hot yoga. In fact, a Finnish study[4] examined the mortality and cardiac events of over 2,000 participants who used dry saunas on a regular basis and found that engaging in two 15-minute sessions, two times a week raised growth hormone release by 500 percent. More importantly, cardiac events dropped nearly 50 percent for those that had a sauna for 15 to 20 minutes, three times a week.

For some people though, a regular sauna can be too hot and suffocating from the intense heat. Also, a traditional sauna, using heated rocks or other heating elements, raises the temperature in the sauna room to about 160 to 200 degrees Fahrenheit, and the shorter wavelengths penetrate the body at a relatively shallow level.

On the other hand, Far Infrared Saunas (FIRS) and their Far Infrared rays create a different experience with better health benefits. A FIRS emits radiant heat which directly heats the body without significantly affecting the surrounding air. This type of heat, usually at temps of 120 to 160 degrees Fahrenheit (49 to 66 degrees Celsius).

This type of heat is often described as gentler and penetrates the skin more deeply. Due to the longer wavelengths and lower temperatures, one can stay in the sauna longer and experience a much deeper sweat and detoxification. In fact, because FIR wavelengths can penetrate at a deeper level, stimulating a greater release of toxins from stored fat, the experts I have studied share that the sweat from an infrared sauna is approximately 75 percent water and 25 percent toxins as compared to 90 percent water and 10 percent toxins from a regular dry sauna.

It's important to note that while saunas can contribute to detoxification, the liver and kidneys are the primary organs responsible for processing and eliminating toxins from the body. Sauna use should be approached with moderation, and individuals with certain health conditions should consult with a healthcare professional before incorporating sauna sessions into their routine. Additionally, staying well-hydrated, as well as supporting electrolytes, is crucial to support the body's natural detoxification processes during and after sauna use.

# Additional Cleansing Tips

## Your lymph system

Optimal lymph flow is crucial for effective body cleansing, as the lymphatic system serves as a key player in removing toxins and waste products from the body. Regular movement, such as rebounding on mini trampolines, proves to be an excellent method for stimulating lymphatic circulation. The rhythmic bouncing encourages the contraction of lymphatic vessels, promoting the flow of lymph throughout the body.

Dry brushing is another technique that enhances lymphatic function by gently exfoliating the skin and encouraging lymphatic drainage. Lymphatic massage, whether performed manually or with the aid of devices like chi machines, can further support the removal of toxins by stimulating lymphatic vessels and nodes. Incorporating these practices into a wellness routine contributes to optimal lymph flow, fostering a comprehensive approach to body cleansing and promoting overall health.

Personally, I've had a monthly lymph massage for years. At times, I've needed them every two weeks. I have found that when I am most consistent with my rebounder and dry brushing, my lymph "check-up" is better—meaning, the level of stagnation is greatly decreased. It's taken a while to get this habit solidified, but now, when I'm at my computer working all day, I set my timer to get up and bounce on that little rebounder for a minute or two. The bonus, it wakes up my brain too. In fact, Jim Kwik, the brain coach, highly recommends this in his book *Limitless*.[5]

## Foods that cleanse

Hippocrates, the renowned ancient Greek physician often hailed as the father of Western medicine, has been given credit for this timeless wisdom: "Let food be thy medicine and medicine be thy food." This profound statement succinctly captures the idea that the food we choose to consume wields the power to either heal or harm. It underscores the direct correlation between our dietary decisions and our overall well-being, echoing a fundamental tenet of holistic medicine.

The significance of this insight cannot be overstated, emphasizing a core principle in holistic medicine. On initial consideration, the quote prompts us to view food as a form of preventive medicine. It serves as a reminder that our dietary choices play a pivotal role in warding off illnesses and fostering good health.

By opting for nourishing ingredients, we fortify our bodies, enhancing our immune systems, boosting energy levels, and bolstering overall resilience. Here are two examples of food groups that indeed can be used as "medicine."

## Cruciferous veggies

Broccoli, cauliflower, and brussel sprouts nourish and support the cleansing pathways in the body, support Glutathione production, and optimize liver function. These superfoods have a chemical called Indole-3-Carbinoles (IC3). These magic molecules help detoxify the nasty xenoestrogens of fake hormones that we are exposed to on a regular basis. However, if you cook these vegetables too much (to the point of smelling them) you will kill the IC3's detoxifying power, so be sure to keep them Al dente.

## Herbs such as rosemary and turmeric

Let's delve into the incredible detoxifying benefits of rosemary and turmeric, focusing on their role in promoting the production of Glutathione.

Firstly, rosemary, with its fragrant aroma and culinary versatility, isn't just a flavorful herb—it also contributes to detoxification. Rosemary contains compounds that support the liver. By aiding the liver in breaking down and eliminating toxins, rosemary indirectly facilitates the creation of Glutathione, our master cellular protector.

Secondly, turmeric is the golden-hued spice renowned for its anti-inflammatory properties. Curcumin, the active ingredient in turmeric, is a powerhouse when it comes to detoxification. It stimulates the production of enzymes that enhance the liver's ability to detoxify harmful substances. Turmeric's connection to Glutathione lies in its capacity to increase the levels of this vital antioxidant in the body.

## Consider This

- What are some sabotaging habits you can transform to promote cleansing of your organs?

- What's a simple "floor" that you can incorporate to support cleansing your body on a daily basis?

# *Nine*

# Cleanse Your Environment

*"The diseases that are today's scourges—*
*diabetes, heart disease, and cancer*
*…are not the effect of a single gene, but of complex interactions*
*among multiple genes and environmental factors."*

~DR. BRUCE LIPTON

Let's talk about some of the environmental factors that you can control to mitigate the negative impact on your genes and increase your chances of experiencing lasting vitality.

## Air

The air you breathe is one of the most important factors to control—both indoors and out. Dust, dust mites, mold, and myco-toxins are toxins that can circulate and create a negative impact on your health. Pet dander, cleaning products, smoking, gas stoves, and high humidity can also wreak significant impact. Short-term symptoms can include dizziness, fatigue, confusion, headaches, nausea, and irritation of the eyes, nose, and throat.

With repeated, long-term exposure, the risks can increase significantly. Prolonged exposure can potentially lead to mood changes and "dirty" your genes, causing respiratory and cardio-vascular diseases, neurological disorders, cancer, and other health conditions. Airborne pollution is also a hazard to pregnant women and young children, increasing the risk of birth defects and developmental problems.

## Improving your indoor air quality

Whether it's dust, dust mites, mold, and mycotoxins, volatile organic compounds (VOC), viruses, or bacteria, improving your indoor air quality is essential for overall well-being. Start by ensuring good ventilation—allow fresh air to circulate by opening windows regularly. Use air purifiers equipped with HEPA filters to capture airborne particles, including allergens and pollutants. Regularly clean and vacuum your home to reduce dust and allergens. Keep humidity levels in check, ideally between 30 to 50 percent, to prevent mold growth. Choose low-VOC (volatile organic compounds) or VOC-free products for cleaning and decorating. Avoid smoking indoors, and consider incorporating indoor plants, known for their air-purifying properties. Regular maintenance of HVAC systems is also crucial.

There are excellent air filters on the market, but the products I recommend and use personally are the April Aire 5000 as a full house air filter, and the IQ-Aire for portable use. I also highly recommend the Ultimatum 1100F ionizer to clear mold, mycotoxins, bacteria, viruses, and MVOCs from your air. Check the Resources section for more information on filters as well as Dr. Dennis's amazing line of mold remediation products.

## Outdoor air

World Health Organization (WHO) data states that 99 percent of the global population breathe air that exceeds healthy guideline limits. Additionally, 2.4 billion people are exposed to dangerous toxins inside the home, such as gas ranges, open fires, kerosine, animal dung, coal, and the mycotoxins from mold. The WHO estimates that almost seven million people around the world die prematurely every year because of air pollution.[1]

This is more than double the previous estimates, making outdoor air pollution one of the leading causes of premature death globally. Its impact on life expectancy is now comparable to poor diets and cigarette smoking. These deaths are a result of the significant impact of air pollution on DNA expression. To quote Ben Lynch, we can make our "good genes dirty."

Most of us think about smog, big diesel motor vehicle exhaust, and outdoor burning or wood smoke as the obvious sources of poor outdoor air quality. However, poor air quality may be closer than you think. Is your yard surrounded by fertilizers or pesticides that contain Glyphosate or other toxins? These too will dramatically "dirty" your genes and increase your risk of negative outcomes. I realize it may be tough to pick up and move, but you can stop the nasty ingredients from being sprayed in your yard and get an air filter for your car.

When I moved into a new home in Atlanta, the lawn was pristine and green, but they were spraying Round Up—the number one marketer for Glyphosate. If you are unfamiliar with the impact of Glyphosate, you can learn more in the Resources section. Let me just say, you do *not* want this in your yard, in your garden, or around your kids or pets. You most definitely do *not* want this on your food! I use extra strength vinegar for the weeds in my yard. It's easy to order on Amazon, and a gallon even comes with a handy dandy sprayer.

I'm fortunate to not have to be out in traffic very often now that I live in Florida, but for my last birthday I got an air filter for my car, and I love it! Check out a simple, portable filter from IQ-Aire in the Resources section. This filter can protect you and your whole family!

# Mold Exposure

The Environmental Protection Agency (EPA) indicates that more than 50 percent of homes and buildings in the U.S. harbor some level of mold. Despite a common perception, mold does not occur only in cities with high humidity.

Many individuals experience heightened reactions, and medical professionals often overlook these symptoms.

Given that we spend about 90 percent of our time indoors, it makes sense that if your living, working, educational, worship, or recreational spaces have experienced any water damage, you could be at risk for mold-related illnesses.

## Understanding mycotoxins

Mycotoxins are toxic compounds generated by specific types of fungi, commonly known as molds, that can thrive on a variety of organic materials such as crops, food items, construction materials, and even in humid indoor environments. These mycotoxins function as naturally occurring secondary metabolites for molds, serving various purposes such as defense against competing organisms. Mycotoxins are potent tools employed by molds to disrupt the equilibrium of our bodies.

Dr. Ritchie Shoemaker, a trailblazer in this field, approximates that around 25 percent of the population possesses a genetic predisposition with specific gene variations that are linked to Glutathione/detoxification pathways. These genetic factors may impact how the body reacts to mycotoxin exposure, potentially rendering individuals susceptible to Chronic Inflammatory Response Syndrome (CIRS), a condition that can arise from mycotoxin exposure.

## Understanding the impact of mold

New stories are reported every day about individuals dealing with the consequences of mold. Take the Smiths, (name changed for privacy) for instance—a family residing in a home plagued by mold. Gradually, they started encountering peculiar symptoms such as hair loss, fatigue, and difficulty concentrating. Subsequent hormone tests unveiled the unsettling truth that mold exposure had disrupted their thyroid hormones and adrenal function, establishing a direct connection between mold and the upheaval of their well-being.

In another scenario, a group of colleagues working in a mold-infested office building observed distressing changes. Escalating mood swings, sleep disturbances, and even irregular menstrual cycles among female colleagues became prevalent. Hormone tests brought to light cortisol imbalances and irregularities in sex hormones, showcasing the subtle but profound impact mold can have on various facets of our health.

Then there's Mary's (name changed for privacy) story, a high school friend who called last year to unveil her own health struggles and those of her partner. Mary battles severe fatigue and now faces lung issues, requiring her to rely on oxygen. Her partner, unfortunately, has been diagnosed with lung cancer. Despite residing in a large city in an exceedingly dry state, a burst pipe in their condo building became the catalyst for their health woes. The remediation team opted to address only a portion of the building, neglecting *their* condo unit. Mary and her partner's health challenges began shortly after the water damage and have progressively worsened over time.

And then there's me. I grappled with profound fatigue and disruptions in my endocrine system for years. My hormone levels plummeted, compelling me to rely on Cortef, a bioidentical cortisol product, as my adrenal glands were incapable of producing sufficient cortisol to meet my daily energy requirements. I constantly felt drained and unwell, struggled with insomnia, felt "wired but tired," gained weight, lost my libido, and suffered from persistent brain fog accompanied by frequent headaches. Collaborating with a functional health provider, I discovered a heavy metal burden, followed by the onset of Epstein-Barre syndrome. Unbeknownst to me, even after addressing these factors over the years, the primary culprit behind my persistent fatigue was severe black mold toxicity. After six intensive months of ozone therapy, the black mold was successfully eradicated. Despite thorough and costly remediation efforts in two residences, every six months new mycotoxins continued to surface in my lab reports. A breakthrough came when my astute doctor recommended a sinus CT scan, revealing the unexpected source of mold—thriving within my own body!

In the summer of 2022, I underwent sinus surgery by Dr. Donald Dennis, an Ear, Nose, and Throat surgeon in Atlanta, Georgia, with over 35 years of surgical experience and extensive graduate training in Biochemistry and Microbiology. This unique background has led to his becoming a global expert in caring for patients with mold sickness. As I went through my post operative healing experience with him, I was shocked one day when he said, "If you go to any pathology department in any city and test the tumors that have been dissected from patients, you will find that almost 80 percent have mold in them." I was startled! And, again, so grateful to get that huge moldy toxic burden out of my head.

Here are some common symptoms of mold toxicity. Can you identify with any of these?

- Abdominal pain and bloating
- Appetite swings
- Chronic fatigue and weakness
- Chronic sinus congestion

- Cognitive impairment
- Cold and flu-like symptoms
- Cough and postnasal drip
- Difficulty concentrating
- Disequilibrium
- Headaches and light sensitivity
- Impotence
- Itchy eyes
- Joint pain
- Metallic taste in mouth
- Nausea and diarrhea
- Red eyes and blurred vision
- Shortness of breath
- Skin sensitivity and rashes
- Watery eyes
- Wheezing

## Electromagnetic Frequencies (EMF) Exposure

We are surrounded by EMF everywhere we go. We have:
- TVs, speakers, gaming consoles, controllers
- Dishwashers, ovens, microwaves, heaters, air conditioners, dehumidifiers
- Wi-Fi routers, computers, tablets, mobile phones, and cordless phones
- Bluetooth devices, such as air pods, fitness trackers, keyboards, wireless mouse, printers, baby monitors
- Amazon Echo or Alexa voice-enabled devices to tie everything together
- There are "smart homes" and entire cities that are "smart cities"

- 5G cell towers
- Smart cars and electric cars

These devices make our lives so convenient in so many ways, yet at what cost?

In his book EMF*D,[2] Dr. Joseph Mercola goes into great depth about what EMFs are and their scientific impact on humans, and he differentiates between ionizing and non-ionizing EMFs. Ionizing EMFs pass through every single tissue in your body! These ionizing frequencies "knock electrons out of the orbit of atoms and turn them into destructive ions that can create damaging free radicals." What does that mean? It means they *damage* your DNA! Non-ionizing EMFs are also dangerous, especially with long-term exposure. Most of the devices listed above are non-ionizing, but still—the cost of long-term exposure to EMFs is huge, no matter the type.

Numerous recent scientific publications[3] *have shown that EMFs affect living organisms at levels well below most international and national guidelines.* According to Dr. Mercola, if you are a 'carb burner,' meaning that you have a high-carb diet, then the impact of EMFs is even worse because they cause even more oxidative free radicals.

Here's just a short list of the some of the major health issues associated with EMFs:

- Anxiety
- Autism—particularly those with a genetic variation (SNP) of CANA1C
- Behavioral problems in children
- Cancer
- Cardiovascular disease
- Chronic fatigue
- Chronic headaches/migraines
- Depression
- Digestion issues

- Emotional issues
- Hyperactivity
- Immune dysfunction
- Infertility
- Insomnia
- Mood disorders

EMF*D goes into significant details on the pathophysiology (disease process), but I want to leave you with simple tips to reduce your EMF exposure.

First, I must address a big issue in our world today—bras and pants with phone pockets. These handy dandy pockets are great for your keys, but many of us are putting our cell phones in them. Oh my! There is already evidence that sperm counts are decreasing in men who put their phones in their front pockets. There is also evidence that cell phones held next to the head are linked to acoustic tumors. Gals, please *do not wear your cell phones in your bras!* While there have been no specific scientific studies yet linking cell phones in the bra with breast cancer, if you read EMF*D, you will absolutely *never* want to wear your phone on your body if it's not in airplane mode.

Here are a few quotes from some prominent breast surgeons:

"Until further data either supports it or disproves it, I would keep cell phones away from the body, in particular the breasts."
~Dr. June Chen, a Breast Cancer Radiologist

"It's as simple as that, and it might save a life, it might avoid a mastectomy, chemotherapy, it's easy enough to do, why take a chance? If there is a risk and we don't find out about it for five or ten years from now, we're going to see a whole cluster of young people with breast cancer."
~Dr. John West, Founder of the Breast Health Awareness Foundation

Now that I've read Mercola's book, I'm grateful that this has been a practice of mine for years.

Second, there are many more simple actions you can take to cut EMF exposure. I get that these can be inconvenient. I get that it's a bit challenging. But you're the one who gets to choose. Incorporating any or all of these suggestions will help to optimize *your* DNA.

- Put your phone in airplane mode when it's not in use.
- Turn off your Wi-Fi when not in use.
- Keep your laptop away from your body—at least 8 inches. Note: Defender Shield is a great company for EMF protection products with laptop shields and cell phone covers. See the Resources section for information.
- Get an ethernet cable or LAN connection for your computer versus Wi-Fi. The Wi-Fi in my home is only on when I use the Peloton; then it goes off again.
- Leave the room when a microwave oven is in use.
- Used wired headphones instead of Bluetooth earbuds.
- Try some grounding essential oils (you can use these via a diffuser, rubbed on the bottom of your feet, or even around your neck in a diffuser necklace).
  - Rose
  - Helichrysum
  - Frankincense
  - Fennel
  - Clove
  - Myrrh
  - Thyme
  - Basil
  - Lavender
  - Grounding—a blend from Young Living

These are just a few of the solutions on the market to help reduce the effects of EMF. We may see more hitting the market in the future. Be sure to check reviews and scientific studies before you purchase however.

## Consider This

- Are you aware of any water damage to a building that you reside in or visit?

- Do you have any mold-related symptoms?

- Do you experience any of the EMF symptoms listed above—if so, how can you eliminate or remediate the effects of EMF around you?

- What are ways that you can transform your environment into a healthier abode?

# *Ten*

# Cleanse Your Mental and Emotional Bodies

*"Inner" healing and changing of belief systems must
take place before the disease is eradicated."*

~ KAROL K. TRUMAN, FEELINGS BURIED ALIVE NEVER DIE

A s you know by now, self-sabotaging thoughts sabotage our
own Epigenetic power. Remember the Epigenetic principles that I shared earlier from Dr. Bruce Lipton, who wrote, "Our thoughts change our biochemistry, which changes the behavior of our cells." In my humble opinion, if you want to achieve the vitality you crave, you must also cleanse self-sabotaging thoughts and emotions.

## Transform Your Thoughts

Dr. Daniel Amen, Dr. Joe Dispenza, and Jim Kwik are a few of my heroes around eliminating self-sabotaging thoughts. First, Dr. Amen's acronym "ANTs" for "automatic negative thoughts," sheds light on the powerful impact of our internal dialogue on our well-being. These automatic negative thoughts act as silent saboteurs, undermining our vitality and influencing our mental and emotional states. Constant exposure to ANTs can contribute to stress, anxiety, and a negative outlook on life.

To eliminate these detrimental thoughts, Dr. Amen suggests employing the "ANT-Killing Technique." This involves becoming aware of the negative thought, labeling it as an ANT, challenging its accuracy, and replacing it with a more positive and constructive thought. By actively recognizing and reshaping automatic negative thoughts, individuals can break free from self-sabotaging patterns and cultivate a more positive mindset conducive to overall health and vitality.

Sometimes we cannot see our own "blind spots." That's why they're called *blind* spots. We may be so used to the tune or tone of our own inner voice that we don't even hear the ANTs. For me, being around people who were "Negative Nellies" or "Energy Vampires" is what helped me to see, hear, and recognize what discordant stinkin' thinkin' looks and feels like. They were leaving abrasive and obvious clues about what their ANTs were. By being around these people, I was finally able to start hearing my own stinkin' thinkin'. The old saying "once you see it, you cannot unsee it" can be very helpful to begin your "ANT-killing" journey.

In the teachings of Dr. Joe Dispenza, a renowned expert in the field of neuroscience and consciousness, he explores the transformative power of our thoughts on the epigenetic dynamics of our bodies. Like Dr. Bruce Lipton, Dr. Dispenza emphasizes that our thoughts have the potential to influence and modify the expression of our genes, shaping the very biology of our existence. Through focused intention, meditation, and the redirection of thought patterns, individuals can activate positive changes at the epigenetic level, influencing health and well-being.

Dr. Dispenza's work emphasizes the notion that by harnessing the power of our minds and cultivating a positive and intentional mental environment, we have the capacity to not only shape our present experience but also contribute to the unfolding of a healthier and more vibrant body, and future. Dr. Dispenza is known for people arriving at his week-long events with very challenging health benefits, and then having miraculous healings in one week—even going from wheelchair bound to walking.

If changing thoughts can do that, how might changing your thoughts impact *your* vitality?

Jim Kwik, the world's master brain coach, teaches in his iconic book *Limitless*[1] that "LIES" are "Limited Ideas Entertained." Think of the LIES as "nothing other than BS (an abbreviation for Belief Systems)" that you may have been telling yourself about your body and how it performs for you, about your mind and how quickly you can or cannot learn, and about your spirit and your capacity to have beautiful relationships. According to the principles of Epigenetics, each of these indeed impact the function or expression of our DNA and our overall capacity to create the vitality that we crave.

## Cleanse Your Emotional Wounds

While this book is not the place to dive into depth on the impact of our relationships or psychosocial impacts on our health—that is, our emotional bodies, I do want to address it here.

Dr. Karol Truman, in her book *Feelings Buried Alive Never Die*, states that: "every feeling, every thought—every emotion we experience sends a message to each cell in our body … each cell is affected either adversely or conversely (negatively or positively). It is not necessary for us to be consciously aware of the message that our cells are receiving. The cells are still being affected. Each DNA and subsequently each cell is impacted by every feeling, every thought … every emotion we experience.[2]

Additionally, Barbara Ann Brennan, a renowned physicist, therapist, healer, scientist, author of *Hands of Light* states that: "… the manifestation of disease takes place when a concept or belief is transmitted (that is, resonated or broadcast) from the mental, emotional, or other areas of our Be-ing into the energy field.[3]

I could continue to quote many experts, but I think you get the point—our emotions impact our DNA. Let's start with the happenings in our childhood.

## Adverse childhood events

Adverse childhood events (ACE) encompass a range of traumatic experiences such as abuse (emotional, verbal, or sexual), neglect, death of a loved one, parental separation or divorce, or witnessing domestic violence. The impact of ACEs extends beyond immediate emotional and psychological consequences—it influences our physiological well-being and even the expression of our genes. Studies have shown that individuals who undergo ACEs may face an increased risk of developing various physical and mental health issues later in life. These events can disrupt the body's stress response system, leading to chronic inflammation, hormonal imbalances, and an elevated risk of conditions like cardiovascular disease and autoimmune disorders.

Furthermore, the effects of ACEs can extend to the realm of Epigenetics, where, as you know, we study any changes in our gene activity that don't involve alterations to the underlying DNA sequence. ACEs can modify the expression of genes associated with the stress response, potentially affecting how the body responds to stressors throughout one's life. Understanding the profound and lasting impact of ACEs on both physiological

*"Being able to feel safe with other people is probably the single most important aspect of mental health; safe connections are fundamental to meaningful and satisfying lives."*

~BESSEL VAN DER KOLK, MD

and epigenetic levels underscores the importance of early intervention, support, and trauma-informed care to mitigate these
long-term effects and promote overall well-being.

*The Body Keeps the Score* by Dr. Bessel van der Kolk is a seminal
work that explores the profound impact of trauma on the body and
mind. Dr. van der Kolk, a psychiatrist and trauma expert, delves into
the intricate ways in which traumatic experiences, whether psychological or relational, can shape our lives. The book emphasizes
that trauma is not just a mental phenomenon; it is stored in the
body and can manifest in physical and psychological symptoms.

One key point is the exploration of how trauma disrupts
the brain's normal functioning, particularly in areas responsible for self-regulation, emotional control, and interpersonal
relationships. Dr. van der Kolk discusses various therapeutic approaches, including neurofeedback, yoga, dancing, and EMDR
(Eye Movement Desensitization and Reprocessing), high-
lighting the potential for healing and recovery. In the years of
doing my healing and recovery work I found that while Cognitive
Behavioral Therapy (CBT) or talk therapy was helpful to unravel
the ANTs, it was EMDR, brain spotting, neurofeedback, and intuitive healing or energy work *combined* with the power of essential
oils that brought about my full healing.

## Trauma throughout our lifespan

Many of the women I have consulted over the years have shared
with me the physical manifestations of the triggering or traumatic events they have experienced. Here's a short list of how their
bodies have kept "the score."

- Brain and Cognitive Function
    - Brain fog
    - Can't concentrate

- – Poor memory
- Heart/Cardiovascular system
  - – Chest pain – Note, some have even experienced "Broken Heart Syndrome" which mimics a heart attack
  - – Pounding chest
- Fatigue
  - – Severe fatigue
- Gut or gastrointestinal system
  - – Constipation
  - – Diarrhea
  - – Indigestion
  - – Nausea
- Lungs
  - – Asthma attacks
  - – I can't breathe
- Musculoskeletal system
  - – Fibromyalgia
- Nervous system
  - – Dizziness
  - – Vertigo
  - – Tinnitus
  - – Severe shivering
  - – Nervous tension in stomach chest, throat with certain sounds
  - – Bothersome lights and sounds
- Reproductive system
  - – Irregular cycles
  - – Heavy bleeding
  - – Bleeding again after years of menopause
- Sleep
  - – Insomnia
  - – Nightmares

# Cleanse Your Limiting Patterns

## Codependency

Codependency is a phrase that has been used for decades, yet there is no *official* diagnosis in the DSM-5 or *Diagnostic and Statistical Manual of Mental Disorders*, 5th edition, published by the American Psychiatric Association. As a result, there are many definitions of what codependency really is. While codependent coping patterns are not your intrinsic personality, many people have developed these traits and coping skills over the years to deal with toxic or challenging situations and relationships. Unfortunately, these patterns that may have been learned as childhood coping skills no longer work as adults. In fact, they are very limiting—limiting our thoughts, beliefs, relationships, and success in multiple areas of our lives. Personally, after being in recovery from codependency for years, the term I have found most helpful is from Ross Rosenberg, PhD, in his book *The Human Magnet Syndrome*. After healing from his own codependency, he has labeled it "Self-Love Deficit Syndrome."[4]

The habitual patterns of rescuing, people-pleasing (which starts as parent-pleasing), enabling, and lack of boundaries inherent in codependency can create a draining cycle that saps the vitality out of anyone. I know this first-hand. Putting others needs before one's own, seeking validation through excessive people-pleasing, and enabling destructive or addictive behaviors can lead to emotional exhaustion and a pervasive sense of fatigue. Been there, done that.

The incessant drive to rescue and fix others often comes at the expense of personal well-being, contributing to a sense of emptiness and burnout. And the absence of clear boundaries further exacerbates this drain, leaving individuals depleted and overwhelmed, even resentful and angry. Breaking free from these life draining habits involves establishing healthy boundaries, prioritizing self-care, and fostering a sense of autonomy. By cultivating a more balanced, differentiated sense of self, you can reclaim your energy and rediscover a sense of fulfillment.

Personally, while I had been doing physical self-care to heal my body for years, it wasn't until I got this message from Dr. Rosenberg that really clarified my need to heal my inner child on a greater level and create healthy boundaries to attain the level of vitality that I want on a spiritual, emotional, mental, and physical level.

To support your emotional and mental reset, I'm sharing my personal SOS list—simple, powerful tools I use to clear and realign.

Find them in the resource section at the back of this book.

## Consider This

- What's a simple habit you can create to transform "ANTs" or "LIES" into positive support thoughts?

- What adverse child events may still be impacting your ability to be your Future-Self?

- What unhealed emotional wounds may be impacting your health and vitality?

- What's a simple floor that you can do to express self-love to yourself every day?

# Section 5

## Optimize Your Cellular Health

## Eleven

# Boost Your Cellular Power
# and Communication

*"The smallest unit of life is the cell.*
*So, if your cells are healthy, you are healthy."*
~MIKE MURPHY, PROFESSOR OF MITOCHONDRIAL REDOX BIOLOGY

D o you or someone you know struggle with fatigue? At least
1.3 percent of American's have been told by their doctor
that they have Chronic Fatigue Syndrome (CFS) (self-reported
as more than six months) — that's more than 4.3 million people.
Many doctors and sleep professionals think almost 90 percent of
those struggling have not been diagnosed. Long-term Covid and
long-term Covid vaccine side effects may also be contributing to
an even greater number.

While it is a multi-factorial issue, this chapter focuses on improving mitochondrial health and cellular communication as they
are critical in overcoming this syndrome as well as revitalizing!

Often, the "treatment" of this nebulous syndrome (CFS) focuses on relieving symptoms, versus getting to the root cause of what
might be causing the mitochondrial dysfunction. Only when your
health care provider asks questions like, "What is inhibiting your
cells making energy?" or "Is there something vital your cell needs
to make energy?" can you begin to make healing headway.

While CFS initially was not my area of specialty, I lived with it
for years. I did not want the energy of that diagnosis defining my
reality or who I was. Thus, I didn't ever identify with the diagnosis

or even speak about it, until I was revitalized and living a healthy life. Now, I'm passionate about helping other women get to the other side of this debilitating syndrome. I will touch on a few basics of cellular energy. Then I will share some more specific information of a few things that are often missed in conventional medicine today, leaving people not only feeling less than vital, but very fatigued!

# Delivering Energy to Your Cells

Adenosine Triphosphate (ATP) is the cellular energy currency that powers various activities within our cells. It's a small molecule with a big job. Think of ATP as a rechargeable battery that stores and delivers energy where it's needed. When our cells need energy to perform tasks like muscle contraction, nerve signaling, or building new molecules, they "spend" that cellular energy currency (which is ATP) by breaking it down. Fortunately, God created ways for ATP to "recharge"—creating a dynamic, continuous cycle of energy within our cells, ensuring that the energy needs of our bodies are met efficiently. Let's examine each one.

### Glutathione

Renowned cardiothoracic surgeon Gregory Brevetti, M.D., stated, "With respect to cellular health, there's air, water, then Glutathione." It's that simple!

As we've discussed, every cell in your body is assaulted by destructive agents—such as free radicals, chemical toxins, heavy metals, and radiation. These destructive agents damage the cell, inhibit optimal function, and accelerate the aging process and the onset/progression of the diseases associated with aging. Again, Glutathione is the master protector of the cell that defends the cell from all these insults. Indeed, it is the master vitality and longevity molecule![1]

Remember, Glutathione has four main functions in protecting each and every cell. It's the

- Master antioxidant
- Master detoxifier
- Master immune system booster
- Master anti-inflammatory

As your body is bombarded with toxins on a daily basis, or has a build up after years of toxic exposure, your Glutathione supply will be focused on detoxifying; thus, you may not have what you need to perform its other functions. This is one of the reasons I encourage my clients to eliminate as many toxins as possible from their diet, their personal care products, and their environment so your Glutathione doesn't have to work so hard in only one area of its four main functions. People with higher Glutathione levels have:

- More energy
- Faster recovery from exercise
- Greater mental clarity and focus
- Less inflammation
- Improved joint function
- Better immune system
- Better sleep
- Longer lives
- Better lives

That's the good news!

The bad news—when exposed to toxins, sleep deprivation, poor food choices, stress, or too much exercise, the decline is even more dramatic.

GSH is also required to break down alcohol in the liver. That daily glass of wine that many consume to relax at night is considered a toxin, and it is therefore accelerating Glutathione decline, increasing oxidative stress, and increasing the uptick of the diseases of aging. These three things are plain physiology or pathophysiology (the disease process), which you can choose or not choose every day.

The more your GSH drops, the faster you experience the diseases of aging—such as decreased stamina, auto-immune disorders, Arthritis, Diabetes, Cancers, Cardiovascular disease, Dementia, Alzheimer's disease, etc.[2] However, the symptoms of GSH decline begins more insidiously—such as feeling fatigued, reduced athletic performance, poor recovery or not "bouncing back" from exercise, brain fog in the afternoon, decreased clarity, toxicity build-up, weakened immune systems, and catching almost every cold that seems to come around.

Yes, aging and death are a part of God's plan; however, many people experience the effects of low Glutathione levels very prematurely. As a result, men and women can suffer health challenges for decades, struggling to maintain some sort of normal function in their various roles. I know firsthand.

It seemed like my health challenges started almost overnight when I turned 42. As I shared earlier, I was challenged with heavy metal toxicity at the time, but then finally discovered Epstein Barre (EBV) and black mold toxicity as well. It took several more years before I found a great DNA test. My suspicions were correct—it revealed that I am completely missing one of my GSH genes. NULL, nada, not there! I have been taking a product with the magical compound RiboCeine ever since. I have eradicated the heavy metals, EBV, and black mold completely.

## What Can You Do?

There are, of course, hundreds of reasons to eat a healthy diet, and supporting your GSH is one of them. Some dietary suggestions to increase your GSH levels naturally may include eating sulfur-rich foods like mushrooms, eggs, fish, and garlic as well as cruciferous veggies like broccoli, kale, and cabbage. While all of these sources may indeed be good, they only raise your GSH minimally, about 20 to 30 percent on average. Eating organic is optimal, as the pesticides and herbicides and other toxins found in our food today can actually use up our Glutathione stores more quickly.

Even whey protein, thought of as an excellent way to increase GSH, has been shown in studies to increase GSH only by 24 percent when taken in high doses of 45 grams a day. If our GSH levels have been dropping 10 percent a decade, we need bigger boosts than that.

The impact is so dramatic, that Glutathione is now the buzz in the medical/scientific community. In fact, there are over 181 thousand medical articles on the critical importance of Glutathione (as compared to 60 thousand articles about Vitamin C), and numerous medical experts are teaching about its benefits at major medical meetings. But why have you not heard about Glutathione before? Because increasing your Glutathione levels has been very difficult and very expensive—*until now.*

I have spent more than 16 years researching the best forms of Glutathione to support my own health and that of my clients. It took 25 years for nine PhDs to crack the biochemical code that brought RiboCeine,[3] a magic compound that helps your body make GSH, to the market. It is the only compound that can optimize endogenous (inside the cell) Glutathione on the market today. In a double-blind, placebo-controlled, human clinical trial, RiboCeine raised serum (blood) GSH levels by 26.6 percent across all study participants (ages 38 to 60 years) and by 64.7 percent in the 51- to 60-year age range. The placebo group experienced a 3.2 percent drop in the same four-week time frame during the holidays. The increase in GSH is quite notable, especially during the holiday season of increased stress, sleep deprivation, and typically a lot of alcohol, too. In addition, to the raise in GSH, the study arm (those that received RiboCeine) also experienced improvement in cerebral blood flow, improved heart rate, improved heart rate variability, and decreased intramuscular fat mass. That is unheard of and, in my opinion, miraculous! See the Resources section for more information.

Whether you are concerned about boosting your immune system, detoxifying your body, reducing inflammation, improving fertility, boosting antioxidant capacity to protect from the diseases of aging, or you just want to feel like you have your mojo back, I invite you to learn more about Glutathione and do what you can to *boost* your levels.

Let me add one thing—a dietary supplement is intended, as the dictionary clarifies, "to supply a deficiency or reinforce." Even though RiboCeine is a scientific breakthrough, it is *not* a "magic bullet." RiboCeine will not override a lousy diet filled with fake, fried, dead, sugar-laden foods, sleep deprivation, a crazy stress load, excessive exercise, lots of alcohol, and exposure to toxins. Managing and eliminating all of these stressors to the body still plays a critical role in your overall Glutathione levels.

However, if you want to increase your vitality and:

- Protect cells, tissues, and organs with superior Glutathione network protection
- Neutralize many types of free radicals
- Promote normal body detoxification
- Help maintain normal body detoxification
- Help maintain healthy joint function
- Promote a healthy immune system
- Support increased energy levels
- Support athletic performance and recovery
- Support the management of inflammation,

then, I highly recommend CellGevity! See the Resources section for more information.

## Magnesium

Magnesium is a crucial mineral that plays a multifaceted role in cellular function and overall health. One of its paramount functions lies in cellular energy production. Magnesium is an essential cofactor for enzymes involved in ATP (adenosine tri-phosphate) synthesis, which remember is the primary energy currency of cells. The presence of magnesium is integral to the phosphorylation reactions that generate ATP, ensuring an efficient energy production process.

Moreover, magnesium is pivotal in neuromuscular transmission and function. It acts as a modulator for ion channels, facilitating the proper flow of ions across cell membranes. This is particularly significant for nerve impulses and muscle contractions, contributing to the overall coordination of the nervous and musculoskeletal systems.

Additionally, magnesium is implicated in maintaining cardiovascular health. It plays a role in regulating vascular tone and is essential for the normal electrical activity of the heart. Ensuring an adequate magnesium intake supports cardiovascular stability by contributing to steady heart rhythm and blood vessel function.

In essence, magnesium's significance extends beyond mere cellular energy production; it encompasses neuromuscular coordination and cardiovascular integrity, making it an indispensable mineral for overall health and well-being.

Magnesium is found in a variety of foods, and incorporating magnesium-rich foods into your diet can be an effective way to ensure an adequate intake. Here are some foods that are good sources of magnesium:

- leafy green vegetables
- nuts and seeds
- whole grains
- legumes

- fish
- avocados
- bananas
- dark chocolate
- dairy products
- Tofu

If you compare my recommended lists of foods to support your cellular health, your hormone health, your heart health, and your brain health throughout these pages, you will notice that these lists repeat many of the same foods. And they all support optimal expression of your DNA. Go figure.

If you need magnesium supplementation, here are some common forms of magnesium:

*Magnesium Citrate:* This form is well-absorbed by the body and is often used for its laxative properties. It's a good option if you are looking to support regular bowel movements. One study found that it may improve blood vessel health in healthy overweight individuals.

*Magnesium Chelate:* This form of magnesium is especially important for muscle building, recovery, and health.

*Magnesium Glycinate:* This form is bound to the amino acid glycine, making it easily absorbed by the body. It is less likely to cause a laxative effect and may be a good choice for those looking to support muscle relaxation and manage stress.

*Magnesium Malate:* This form is the most bioavailable form of magnesium. It is bound to malic acid, which is involved in energy production. It may be beneficial for individuals seeking support for muscle pain and fatigue.

*Magnesium Oxide:* While this form has a high magnesium content, it is less bioavailable than other forms. It is often used as a laxative and may be suitable for individuals with constipation.

*Magnesium Taurate:* This form combines magnesium with the amino acid taurine and is the form of magnesium best for your heart and supporting normal blood pressure.

*Magnesium L-Threonate:* This form is believed to penetrate the blood-brain barrier more effectively, making it a potential choice for those looking to support cognitive function.

*Magnesium Orotate:* While helpful for the heart, this form of magnesium is believed to be the best form for metabolic improvements. It's a great option for athletes who want optimized recovery, energy, and performance.

It's important to note that the body's response to magnesium can vary among individuals, and the best form for one person may not be the same for another. Remember, I'm a big believer in bio-individualized care and treatment. Factors such as absorption rate, potential side effects, and the specific health goals you have in mind should be considered. If you have any concerns or pre-existing health conditions, it's advisable to consult with a healthcare professional before starting magnesium supplementation. For supplement recommendations see the Resources section.

## Coenzyme Q10

Coenzyme Q10 (CoQ10), also known as ubiquinone, is a superhero inside our cells. In fact, this vital compound found in the mitochondria—the energy factory of cells—plays a central role in the production of adenosine triphosphate (ATP), the cell's primary energy source. Basically, CoQ10 reminds me of the fireman or stoker that worked alongside the engineer of old steam engine trains. The engineer might direct the train, but the stoker ensured that the coal was put in the engine, so the train can have adequate fuel and be propelled down the track.

Beyond its crucial role in energy production, CoQ10 also serves as a potent antioxidant, protecting cells from oxidative damage by the nasty scavenging oxygen free radicals. While the body can synthesize CoQ10 (ubiquinone) to ubiquinol inside the cell, its levels decline with age or due to certain medical conditions. Ubiquinol is present in just about everything we eat, yet you would need to eat a significant amount of food to get the recommended 100 mg per day. Additionally, some people are born with a genetic mutation in the NQO1 gene, and thus cannot convert CoQ10 (ubiquinone) to the active important form, ubiquinol. Thus, these people definitely need to take ubiquinol (*vs. ubiquinone or Co-Q10*) as a supplement. See the Resources section.

The additional bonus of supplementing with 100 to 300 mg of ubiquinol daily is that is has been shown to:
- Support endothelial function (the lining of your vessels)[4]
- Prevent cardiovascular events
- Decrease LDL cholesterol[5]

Note—Statin drug therapy, widely used globally, is known through clinical trials to significantly reduce ubiquinol,[6] thus supplementation is highly recommended to protect your heart *and* your cellular energy supply.

## Hydration

Hydration is so important to our vitality that I mention it in Chapter 8 about cleansing our organs and in Chapter 18 when discussing Your Daily Vitals for vitality. It's also important to your cellular energy, so I address it here, too.

When it comes to water and its capacity to energize your cells, I like to think of Niagara Falls or the Iguazu Falls in Brazil. You can think of any waterfall really, and consider the powerful energy that is emitted from these water sources. In the United

States alone, Niagara Falls provides 2.6 million kilowatts of clean electricity, making it New York state's biggest electrical producer.

Whenever I feel sluggish, I know that I need water—good, clean, water. Our brains are ¾ water[7] and as Jim Kwik teaches, our brains can lose up to a pound of water when we sleep. So, if you want your brain to be bright and sharp first thing in the morning, drink a big glass of water. If you add Himalayan Sea salt or ELMT, you will also provide an extra spark of energy to your adrenal glands. See the Resources section for more information.

## Omega 3 fatty acids

For years, the nucleus was taught as the brain of the cell directing all of the important cellular functions. Well, now we know other- wise. It is the cell membrane that is actually the "brain" of the cell, because it is critical for healthy cellular communication and takes charge of what passes in and out of the cell. To support a healthy cell membrane, start by increasing Omega 3 Fatty acids, like wild caught salmon, sardines, and chia and flax seeds.

# Cellular Receptivity

Think of a cell phone. We know we can charge our cell phone battery, but if we are in an area that has poor reception, then we may not be able to communicate. It takes the power *and* the good reception to get the conversation delivered. When our phone has all four bars fully functioning, there is a good chance that the per- son on the other end will hear our message, if *they* also have four bars. Even if your cell phone battery is charged, if you don't have enough bars, the message will not go through.

It's the same with your hormones.

Hormones are messenger proteins, and often their message is not heard because the communication is not being heard at the cellular level. This can be referred to as poor cell receptor function or poor cellular receptivity.

Poor cellular receptivity occurs when the cells in the body don't respond well to the signals sent by the hormones. Hormones are chemical messages produced within various glands in the body that help regulate many physiological processes, including growth and development, metabolism, and reproductive functions.

When a hormone is released into the blood stream, it travels to specific cells in the body and bind to the receptor on the surface or inside the cell, similar to a lock and key. The binding triggers a series of chemical reactions inside the cell, leading to a specified response.

However, if the cells don't have enough hormone receptors, if they are clogged and don't work, they may not respond well to the hormone signal. This can lead to imbalances and various health problems.

For example, in insulin resistance, the cells in the body don't respond well to the hormone insulin. Due to the constant barrage of sugar/glucose, the body has had to continuously pump insulin to lower the blood sugar. After a while, the cells no longer respond or become resistant to the insulin. This, in turn, leads to high blood sugar levels and eventually diabetes.

Another example is thyroid hormone resistance, where the cells in the body don't respond well to the thyroid hormone. This causes symptoms of fatigue, weight gain, and dry skin, among others.

There are many other examples of hormonal disorders that can be caused by poor cellular receptivity, but the underlying mechanism is essentially the same—the cells in the body are not responding properly to the hormone signals they receive, leading to symptoms.

How many women do you know who have had their "parts" taken out because they were supposedly "causing" hormonal symptoms or health challenges?

Sadly, over 600,000 women annually[8] have their parts taken out to *solve the problem* or to relieve the symptoms, and yet they still find themselves to be without ideal vitality. Often, what's truly missing is proper cellular communication as well as poor cellular receptivity. Thus, a focus on ascertaining why the body is not 'functioning' optimally is the brilliance of "functional" medicine.

## Cofactors for good cellular communication

Nutrition and the important "cofactors" that good nutrition provide are critical for cellular communication. Cholesterol is at the top of the complicated sex (steroid) hormone cascade. It then converts to pregnenolone, which then converts to progesterone. Progesterone—considered the "life giving" hormone—converts to the androgens (testosterone and DHEA) as well as the estrogens and cortisol. For any of these biochemical conversions to take place, specific phytonutrients are required as cofactors. Guess where those phytonutrients come from? Greens! We need greens to achieve hormonal harmony!

I see so many women who are incredibly symptomatic with hormonal imbalance, in part because their diet is so poor and they are not giving their body (and their hormonal cascade) the nutrition it needs to perform its magic. We'll discuss hormonal harmony in detail in Chapter 14. But for now, let me share a story about when a lack of greens (a nutritional cofactor necessary for optimal hormone function) disrupted my cellular communication.

When I was first diagnosed with Leaky Gut syndrome, and as a result a broken blood brain barrier (also known as "Leaky

Brain syndrome"), I was told I needed to be on a gluten free, dairy free diet for a year. Well, a trip to Italy was on the calendar, and I did not want to be in Italy with the amazing breads, pasta, and gelato on those dietary restrictions. So after the year was up, when my body had healed significantly, I was given the freedom to go and to eat anything I wanted! I did enjoy the bread, and some pasta, and the gelato. Yes, this girl even indulged in the sugar of gelato!

Here's where the challenge was—I was used to eating plentiful greens every single day. But in Italy, I could not find greens anywhere. (Well, except the amazing pesto.) Within four days, I was hot flashing day and night—all night. Wow. What I had been teaching my clients for years—from didactic, textbook knowledge—was now hitting me like a brick wall. Finding greens all of a sudden became an urgent matter. Needless to say, I do *not* travel without my greens now. See the Resources section for my recommended product created by Anna Cabeca, M.D.

## More examples of poor cellular communication

If we continue with the cell phone analogy, one bar of signal will leave you feeling symptomatic. If you have four bars, then the message can get through the intricate communication from your brain to your hormone-sensitive tissues. When communication is clear like this, you are blessed with vitality, a clear mind, and all the benefits of happy hormones all over the body!

The challenge is there are *many* things that junk up our cell receptors. These chemicals and toxins are often called:

- **Hormone Disrupters** – they disrupt normal hormone signaling
- **Endocrine Disrupters** – The Endocrine system is the name of the system in the body

that makes the hormones. Thus these toxins *disrupt* the normal function of this system:

- **Xenoestrogens** – Xeno means foreign, thus these are synthetic foreign estrogens
- **Hormone Mimickers** – these toxins look like real hormones and try to *mimic* their effect
- **Environmental estrogens** – obviously, these toxins are found in the air we breathe and the water we drink
- **Obesogens** – these toxins are stored in fat and are like magnets to fat

They are also everywhere in our modern worlds, including many of the things we've discussed in Chapter 9:

- the air we breathe (*molds, ammonia, glyphosate*)
- the water we drink (*chlorine, ammonia, fluoride, petroleum*)
- the food we eat (*such as preservatives and the artificial food coloring known as FD&C Red No. 3 and bovine growth hormones, propyl gallate and 4-hexylresorcinol*)
- the personal care products we use (*sodium laurel sulfate, chlorine, benzophenone, phthalates, parabens*)
- the cleaning products we use (*chlorine, triclosan, ammonia, sodium hydroxide, perchloroethylene or* PERC)
- the yard care products (*glyphosate, organophosphate pesticides*)

Do any of those sound like something you want getting in the way of your cellular communication? I say absolutely not!

As we discussed in Chapter 8, cleansing the toxins from your cells and your body is the first step toward enhancing cellular communication. The next step is incorporating what I call the Daily Vitals of breath, nourishment, hydration, movement, and sleep, which we'll discuss in Chapter 18. Specific Nutraceuticals, homeopathy, and minerals also play a role in improving cellular communication. See the Resources section.

# *Consider This*

- What are some ingredients in your environment or personal care products that might be clogging up your cellular communication?

- What products can you swap out for clean and green ones?

- What other things can you add to optimize your cellular communication and energy?

- What's a simple "floor" that you can incorporate to improve your cellular function and cellular receptivity?

# *Twelve*

# Biohacks for Cellular Health

*Biohacking—"The art and science of changing*
*the environment around you and inside you, so you*
*have more control over your own biology."*
~DAVE ASPREY

These biohacking modalities are what I have used personally and recommended to my clients for years. Therapies that may have been "leading edge" or "cutting edge" when I began using them twenty years ago are now researched and common in the world of biohacking and longevity medicine.

## Biohacking Modalities

### Glutathione

I've shared information on Glutathione in chapter 8 and chapter 11, illustrating just how important this supplement is. Yet, I would be remiss if I did not mention Glutathione as a primary biohacking tool.

As stated earlier, the three most important things your cells need to optimize cellular health are: 1) air, 2) water, and 3) Glutathione. With that said, I feel the first step in Biohacking should be to augment or support our Glutathione levels as we age. See the Resources section for more information about the product I use and recommend.

## Grounding

Grounding, also known as earthing, refers to the practice of connecting with the Earth's natural energy by direct physical contact with the ground. This involves activities such as walking barefoot on grass, soil, or sand, but there are also grounding devices available that conduct the Earth's electrical charge. Proponents of grounding believe that it offers a range of health benefits, both physiological and psychological.

One key benefit of grounding is its potential to reduce inflammation in the body. The Earth carries a negative electric charge, and proponents argue that direct contact with the ground allows individuals to absorb electrons, which can neutralize positively charged free radicals and reduce inflammation. Inflammation is associated with various chronic health conditions, and some studies suggest that grounding may have a positive impact on inflammatory markers.[1]

Another potential advantage of grounding is improved sleep quality. In our modern lifestyle, characterized by constant exposure to electronic devices and artificial lighting, circadian rhythms and sleep patterns can be disrupted. Grounding is believed to help reset the body's internal clock, promoting better sleep and addressing issues such as insomnia.[2] Some individuals report experiencing deeper and more restful sleep after incorporating grounding practices into their daily routine.

Lastly, proponents of grounding suggest that it may contribute to stress reduction and emotional well-being. Connecting with nature and the Earth's energy is thought to have a calming effect on the nervous system, potentially lowering cortisol levels and promoting a sense of balance and tranquility. While scientific research on grounding is ongoing and not yet conclusive, many individuals find the practice to be a simple and accessible way to enhance their overall well-being.

A friend, I'll call her Janice, was living in a foreign country for a few years. While the home she was living in was lovely, she was unable to sleep. In fact, she had not slept more than four hours per night for 18 months. She was exhausted—physically, emotionally, and mentally. She had tried everything under the sun to aid her sleep, and nothing was working. When she came back to the states for a short visit, I finally found out about her incredible sleep disorder. Immediately I recommended a grounding sheet. It worked! Within a matter of a week, she was sleeping through the night. See the Resources section for my recommendations.

There's a reason that I walk on the beach often. There's a reason that I like to walk barefoot on the grass. But when I can't or don't, I am very grateful for my grounding sheet. I have a spare one in my luggage that accompanies me on all travel.

## PEMF

PEMF stands for Pulsed Electromagnetic Field Therapy, and it's a form of energy medicine that involves the use of electromagnetic fields to positively influence the body's functions and promote overall well-being. PEMF involves the application of electromagnetic fields with specific frequencies and intensities to the body. These pulsing electromagnetic fields are thought to interact with the body's cells, tissues, and organs, influencing cellular processes and promoting balance. PEMF devices can vary in terms of their strength, frequency, and application methods.

The basic principle behind PEMF is that the electromagnetic fields applied resonate with the natural frequencies of the body's cells. This resonance is believed to enhance cellular function by promoting optimal energy production, improving nutrient exchange, and supporting waste elimination. By positively influencing cellular processes, PEMF may contribute to overall vitality.

### Energy production and mitochondrial health

PEMF is thought to support cellular energy production, particularly in the mitochondria—the energy-producing organelles within cells. By optimizing mitochondrial function, PEMF may enhance the body's capacity for energy generation. Improved cellular energy metabolism is associated with increased vitality and overall well-being.[3]

### Stress reduction and relaxation

PEMF has been suggested to have stress-reducing effects on the body. The application of electromagnetic fields may help modulate the nervous system, promoting a state of relaxation. Chronic stress is known to contribute to various health issues. By helping the body manage stress, PEMF may indirectly contribute to longevity and overall health.

### Joint health and recovery

Some biohackers and individuals interested in longevity explore PEMF for its potential benefits on joint health and recovery. The therapy may aid in reducing inflammation, supporting the healing of soft tissues,[4] and improving overall joint function.[5] This can be particularly relevant for individuals dealing with musculoskeletal issues or those seeking to optimize physical performance.

### Sleep quality and circadian rhythms

PEMF has been studied for its potential impact on sleep quality and circadian rhythms. Exposure to specific electromagnetic frequencies may influence the body's internal clock, promoting better sleep patterns. Since quality sleep is a key factor in overall health and longevity, PEMF's role in supporting sleep is of interest to biohackers and health enthusiasts.

## Rebounder/trampoline

A rebounder, or mini-trampoline, has gained popularity in health and fitness circles for its potential to contribute to overall well-being and longevity,[6] making it a noteworthy element in the realm of biohacking. The use of a rebounder involves performing various exercises, such as bouncing, jogging, and jumping, on a small, spring-loaded trampoline.

Almost twenty years ago, when I was introduced to the rebounder, I was astonished to see the health benefits associated with it. In fact, a family member who has had years of physical health challenges and could barely walk up the stairs began to gently use the "Celleriser" (*see the Resources section*) every day with a bar to hold on to. We were all shocked to watch her energy, stamina, and leg strength improve to the point of no longer needing support up and down the stairs. Almost twenty years later and well into her nineties, she has more stamina, strength, and zip than she had for years!

Personally, I think that rebounding is one of the most important exercises we can do. I often use mine with mini weights, will bounce and repeat my daily affirmations, or just dance and have a great time. When I'm at my desk working, I set a timer for every 16 to 20 minutes and then get up and do the mini-tramp to stimulate my lymph and the blood flow to my brain. Check out the following additional benefits.

### Cellular exercise and detoxification

Rebounding provides a unique form of exercise that involves repetitive, controlled movements against gravity. This action stimulates every cell in the body, promoting cellular health and enhancing the efficiency of various bodily systems. The up-and-down motion of rebounding supports the lymphatic system, which plays a crucial role in detoxification. The rhythmic bouncing helps move lymph fluid through the lymphatic vessels, facilitating the removal of waste and toxins from the body.

## Cardiovascular health and improved circulation

Regular use of a rebounder offers a low-impact cardiovascular workout that can improve heart health and circulation. The gravitational forces experienced during rebounding enhance blood flow and oxygenation, promoting a healthy cardiovascular system. This type of exercise can be particularly beneficial for individuals who may have joint issues or find high-impact exercises challenging.

## Bone density and joint support

Rebounding is considered a weight-bearing exercise, which is crucial for maintaining and improving bone density. The gentle impact on the bones during rebounding helps stimulate bone formation, supporting skeletal health. Additionally, the controlled nature of rebounding minimizes stress on joints, making it an accessible and joint-friendly exercise option for people of various fitness levels.[7]

## Stress reduction and improved mental health

Exercise, including rebounding, is well-known for its positive impact on mental health. The rhythmic bouncing can be a fun and enjoyable activity, releasing endorphins and reducing stress levels. Incorporating rebounding into a biohacking routine may contribute to an overall sense of well-being and help manage stress, which is crucial for optimizing health and longevity.

## Lymphatic pumping and immune system support

The lymphatic system is a key component of the immune system, and rebounding acts as a natural lymphatic pump. The bouncing motion helps move lymph fluid, facilitating the circulation of immune cells and enhancing the body's ability to defend against infections and illnesses.[8] Supporting the lymphatic system through rebounding may play a role in strengthening the immune response.[9,10]

## Heat and cold therapy

Hot and cold therapies, often associated with practices like sauna use and cold plunges, offer a range of physiological benefits that support biohacking. These contrasting therapies, known as thermotherapy and cryotherapy, respectively, can be powerful tools to optimize various aspects of physical and mental well-being.

I began my "thermotherapy" or infrared sauna use almost twenty years ago when I found out about my severe heavy metal toxicity and was told this therapy could help with detoxification. It has become a wonderful habit of self-care where I can listen to beautiful solfeggio music or mediate.

Cold therapy on the other hand—I'm just warming up to the idea. I hate being cold, but I know the biohacking benefits are significant. So even this girl, while not jumping in ice baths yet, is gradually increasing the time I spend under the cold water, while the shower is warming up. Since the majority of disease is associated with inflammation and toxicity, I am totally up for mastering this cold therapy, too.

Below are some of the physiological benefits of both.

### Hot therapy (sauna use)

Sauna therapy involves exposing the body to elevated temperatures, typically in a dry or infrared sauna. The benefits of hot therapy include:

*Detoxification:* Saunas induce sweating, which is a natural process for eliminating toxins from the body. Sweating helps cleanse the skin and can contribute to the removal of heavy metals and other substances through the pores.[11]

*Improved Circulation:* Exposure to heat in saunas promotes vasodilation—the expansion of blood vessels—leading to improved circulation. This can enhance oxygen and nutrient delivery to tissues, supporting overall cardiovascular health.[12,13]

*Muscle Relaxation and Recovery:* The heat from saunas helps relax muscles, alleviating tension and promoting recovery. Regular sauna use can be particularly beneficial for individuals engaged in physical training or those with muscle stiffness.[14]

*Stress Reduction:* Sauna sessions can induce a state of relaxation, leading to reduced stress levels. The release of endorphins, often referred to as the "feel-good" hormones, contributes to an improved mood and mental well-being.

## Cold therapy (cold plunges)

Cold therapy involves exposure to cold temperatures, often through methods like cold plunges or ice baths. The benefits of cold therapy include:

*Anti-Inflammatory Effects:* Cold exposure triggers vasoconstriction, the narrowing of blood vessels, leading to a reduction in inflammation. This can be particularly beneficial for athletes dealing with exercise-induced inflammation or individuals with chronic inflammatory conditions.[15]

*Enhanced Recovery and Muscle Repair:* Cold therapy may accelerate the recovery process by reducing muscle soreness and promoting efficient muscle repair. It is commonly used by athletes to facilitate quicker recovery between training sessions.

*Increased Metabolism and Caloric Expenditure:* Exposure to cold temperatures can stimulate brown adipose tissue (BAT), which burns calories to generate heat. Cold therapy may contribute to increased metabolic activity and, in some cases, support weight management efforts.

*Mental Alertness and Stress Adaptation:* Cold exposure is thought to activate the sympathetic nervous system, leading to increased alertness and mental clarity. Cold plunges can also act as a form of stress adaptation, helping individuals become more resilient to stressors over time.[16]

Integrating both hot and cold therapies into a biohacking routine, known as contrast therapy, allows individuals to harness the benefits of both temperature extremes. Alternating between hot and cold exposures can enhance circulation, support detoxification, and optimize the body's adaptive responses. As with any biohacking strategy, it's crucial to consider individual tolerance levels and consult with a healthcare professional if there are any underlying health concerns.

## Stem cell therapy

Stem cell (SC) therapy is gaining attention in the realm of biohacking for its potential to enhance health, regeneration,[17] and overall well-being. While I've been intrigued for years, and even started some therapy a few years ago, I was unaware of the power of SCs and how effective they could be in regenerative medicine until summer of 2023. That's when I heard Christian Drapeau, neurophysiologist and author or *Cracking the Stem Cell Code*,[18] speak at a biohacking conference. My jaw nearly hit the floor when I saw the before and after pictures of patients with severe cardiomyopathy (heart failure). These patients, on transplant lists for such severe heart failure, were taken off the transplant lists and beginning to live normal healthy lives because of stem cell therapy—in this case supporting the migration of stem cells daily throughout the body.

CREATE THE VITALITY YOU CRAVE

Drapeau summarizes that stem cells are defined as "cells with the unique capacity to self-replicate throughout the entire life of an organism and can differentiate into various cell types in the body." Embryonic stem cells (ESCs) that are extracted from an embryo within five to ten days can differentiate into bone cells, heart cells, liver cells, and nervous cells. While extraordinary, ESCs are associated with considerable ethical concerns, thus more focus and scientific research is now associated with Adult Stem Cells (ASCs). The role of ASCs, most predominantly found in the bone marrow and blood, is to maintain and repair the tissues in which they are found. Much of Drapeau's work has been focused on the importance of stimulating the mobilization of the ASCs to migrate to the tissues that need repair.

Here are more in-depth insights into the benefits of stem cell therapy as it relates to biohacking.

## Tissue regeneration and repair

Stem cells have the unique ability to transform into different cell types, and this property is harnessed in stem cell therapy to promote tissue regeneration and repair. Biohackers may explore stem cell interventions to address issues related to joint health, muscle injuries, and other degenerative conditions. By injecting or introducing stem cells into targeted areas, the therapy aims to stimulate the natural healing processes of the body.

## Anti-aging effects

The regenerative potential of stem cells is often associated with anti-aging benefits.[19] As the body ages, the ability of tissues and organs to repair and regenerate diminishes.[20] Stem cell therapy, in theory, could counteract this decline by introducing new, functional cells to replace damaged or aging ones.[21] Those interested in optimizing longevity and slowing the aging process may explore stem cell interventions as part of their anti-aging toolkit.

### Cognitive enhancement

While research in this area is still in its early stages, there is growing interest in the potential cognitive benefits of stem cell therapy. The idea is that stem cells could contribute to the repair of neural tissues and enhance cognitive performance, potentially addressing issues related to neurodegenerative conditions or age-related cognitive decline.

### Enhanced recovery from injuries

Athletes and individuals engaged in intense physical activities may turn to stem cell therapy to accelerate the recovery process from injuries. Whether it's a sports-related injury or general wear and tear on joints and muscles, the regenerative properties of stem cells may support faster healing and tissue repair, allowing anyone to optimize their physical performance.

### Immune system modulation

Stem cells can modulate the immune system, influencing its activity and responsiveness. Those interested in immune system optimization may explore the beneficial effects of stem cells that can potentially contribute to a more balanced and efficient immune response.

### Hair regrowth and aesthetics

Stem cell therapy is being explored as a potential treatment for hair loss and aesthetic purposes.[22] Biohackers interested in optimizing their appearance may consider stem cell interventions to stimulate hair follicle regeneration and improve skin quality.

While research in this area is ongoing, early findings suggest potential benefits in the field of aesthetics. Sign me up!

It's important to note that while the potential benefits of stem cell therapy are promising, the field is still evolving, and research continues to explore the safety and efficacy of different approaches. Additionally, ethical considerations and regulatory frameworks surrounding stem cell therapy should be carefully considered. As with any biohacking intervention, individuals should consult with qualified healthcare professionals and stay informed about the latest developments in stem cell research.

## Ozone therapy

Ozone therapy is an alternative medical treatment that involves the introduction of ozone, a molecule consisting of three oxygen atoms, into the body for therapeutic purposes. Once the ozone is in the body, the molecule breaks down into three free floating oxygen molecules that are now able to do magic throughout the body.

In January of 2010, I was coming down my stairs early one morning and slipped. I fell down 14 steps and tore several tendons and ligaments in my ankle. The great news, I was literally on my way to the integrative medicine clinic for a check-up. Within a few hours of the injury, I was given an ozone injection into my ankle tissues.

All I knew of ozone therapy at the time was the ozone in our atmosphere. I had an additional injection, and did physical therapy, and in six weeks was back in my five-inch heels. Yes, I still wear five-inch heels on the weekend.

When I was diagnosed with severe levels of black mold toxicity, I finally attended a three-day medical conference on ozone therapy. I was astonished at the benefits. After purchasing an ozone generator, I proceeded to do ozone treatments at home, every other day. In six months, I was elated to find that the black mold levels were at zero! Gone. I continue to use ozone therapy as a regular biohacking practice.

Here's a sample of the longevity and biohacking properties of ozone therapy.

### Immune system modulation

Ozone therapy is believed to modulate the immune system, enhancing its ability to combat infections, viruses, and bacteria.[23] Ozone has antimicrobial properties and may stimulate the production of immune cells, such as white blood cells (WBCs). By optimizing immune function, biohackers may aim to bolster their body's natural defenses against pathogens, potentially reducing the risk of illness.[24,25] Personally, Epstein Barre and black mold sent my WBCs plummeting. Ozone therapy brought them back up to healthy levels while I was in the process of killing off the toxins.

### Antioxidant effects

Ozone therapy is thought to have antioxidant effects, helping to counteract oxidative stress in the body. Oxidative stress, caused by an imbalance between free radicals and antioxidants, is implicated in aging and various chronic diseases. Many providers that recommend ozone therapy do so to help heal even cardiovascular disease.

### Improved oxygen utilization and wound healing

Ozone therapy is believed to enhance the utilization of oxygen in the body's cells. By facilitating the delivery of oxygen to tissues and improving cellular oxygenation, biohackers may aim to optimize metabolic processes. Improved oxygen utilization is crucial for energy production and overall cellular function, potentially contributing to increased vitality and longevity.

Part of the benefit of the improved oxygen utilization is enhanced wound healing. As a very young nurse, I worked in nursing homes and had to change the bandages of those with severe bed sores. It could take months or even longer for these wounds to heal. The dressings changes were excruciating for patients. As I sat there in this medical conference, I was astonished to see that wounds that had not been healing in a year began to heal within a week of ozone therapy. I too have had significant wound healing, after cutting my finger a full skin thickness deep. In one week of using ozonated oil, my finger was completely healed.

## Mitochondrial support

As you know by now, the mitochondria play a key role in energy production. Ozone therapy is thought to support mitochondrial function by promoting oxygen delivery and reducing oxidative stress. Biohackers interested in optimizing their cellular energy metabolism may explore ozone therapy as a potential strategy for mitochondrial support.[26]

## Detoxification and anti-inflammatory effects

Ozone therapy is suggested to have detoxification properties, aiding in the elimination of toxins from the body. Additionally, it may have anti-inflammatory effects, potentially reducing inflammation, which is implicated in many chronic diseases. Biohackers seeking to support their body's natural detoxification processes and mitigate chronic inflammation may consider ozone therapy as part of their biohacking toolkit.

## Longevity principles

While the direct link between ozone therapy and longevity is an area of ongoing research, some biohackers are drawn to the idea that its immune-modulating, antioxidant, and cellular support properties may contribute to overall well-being and increased lifespan. After all, I want my clients to have their vitality equal their longevity. Ozone therapy is one practice that I have incorporated to do just that.

It's essential to note that the use of ozone therapy is a subject of debate in the medical community, and potential risks and side effects should be carefully considered. Biohackers interested in exploring ozone therapy should do so under the guidance of qualified healthcare professionals who can provide informed advice based on individual health considerations.

## Biohacking for Life

In summary, while traditional medicine may not use these modalities, there are providers all over the world that have been using them and rigorously studying their healing properties for decades. You may need to talk with your individual provider, yet from my own personal experience, these therapies have been so beneficial.

Biohacking is not just for the rich and famous! For a quick-reference guide of simple, free strategies, check out the resource section at the back of the book.

## *Consider This*

- *From the information above, are there simple things that you feel you can add to your life to increase your longevity and vitality?*

- *If you could add one new biohacking therapy to your health routines, which one feels like a good fit for you?*

# Section 6

## *The Power of Balance*

*Thirteen*

# Balance Your
# Gut-Brain Connection

*"Your gut has capabilities that surpass all your
other organs and even rival your brain."*

~EMERAN MAYER, MD

Most of us have been told to "trust your gut" or "listen to your gut." Science now shows there is indeed a connection between our gut and our brain, now known as the gut-brain axis.[1] This axis serves as a two-way street, linking our central nervous system (CNS) with our enteric nervous system (ENS), which oversees the extensive microbial community[2] in our gut. This link-up, via the Vagus nerve, essentially connects the emotional and cognitive hubs in our brain with our gut's microbiome.

Research across multiple fields, from neuroscience to gastroenterology, has revealed just how profound this relationship is for our overall health and happiness. It turns out that disruptions in this gut-brain axis can throw a wrench into the works, contributing to a whole host of issues. Mood disorders like depression and anxiety,[3] neurodegenerative conditions such as Alzheimer's disease,[4] and pesky gastrointestinal problems like irritable bowel syndrome (IBS) can result from disruptions in your gut-brain axis.

This is why it's become increasingly important to explore ways to keep your gut microbiome in balance. After all, nurturing a harmonious environment in your gut isn't just about dodging tummy troubles—it's about looking after both your physical well-being and your emotional and mental health.

## Balance Your Gut Microbiome

The gut microbiome refers to all the microbes in your intestines, which are organs that are crucial for your health in addition to your cleansing organs that we discussed in Chapter 8. There are more *bacterial* cells in your body than *human* cells. In fact, there are roughly 40 trillion bacterial cells in your body and only 30 trillion human cells. That means you are more bacteria than human! What's more, there are up to 1,000 species of bacteria in the human gut microbiome, and each of them plays a different role in your body. Most of them are extremely important for your health, while others may cause disease.[5]

In his landmark book, *Super Gut*, Dr. William Davis[6] states "no body system is immune to the effects of the monster we have created called the modern human microbiome." Wow! No body system? What we have created, especially in the last 100 years, is what Dr. Davis refers to as "Frankenbelly."

Recent studies[7] suggest that the intestinal microbiome, the "Frankenbelly" coined by Davis, plays an important role in modulating risk of several chronic diseases, including inflammatory bowel disease, Crohn's disease, constipation, obesity, type 2 diabetes, cardiovascular disease, colon cancer, and even depression and despair. Additionally, studies examining the composition and role of the intestinal microbiome[8] in different disease states have uncovered associations with inflammatory skin diseases such as psoriasis and atopic dermatitis[9], autoimmune arthritis, fibromyalgia, fatty liver disease, Parkinson's disease, Alzheimer's disease dementia, restless leg syndrome, and even premature deliveries.

Dr. Davis highlights research from anthropologists and epidemiologists that reveals that in countries where they still have a primitive diet, they have healthy microbiomes that include microbes that are not "ghosts of microbes past"—such as in our Western world due to our toxic, sugar laden, high carb, processed diets. In fact, "consumption of refined sugar triggers rapid changes in the intestinal bacterial species present…yielding to irritable bowel syndrome within *days* of increased sugar intake."[10]

Davis goes into extraordinary depth in his book in detailing what to avoid to optimize your gut microbiome. It also includes specific Super Gut recipes to support and grow healthy microbiome.

Here's a short list of what he recommends to amend and prepare our "garden" to grow optimal bowel flora:

- **Avoid sugar** – lots of sugar "virtually guarantees" a set up for inflammatory bowel disease. Choose monk fruit sweetener or stevia.
- **Avoid synthetic non-caloric sweeteners** – including aspartame, sucralose, or saccharine. Choose monk fruit sweetener or stevia.
- **Banish processed foods that contain emulsifying agents** – emulsifiers make things creamy—like peanut butter and ice cream—but they degrade the mucus lining, cause changes in the bowel flora, and increase intestinal permeability. Hello gas, bloating, pain, and inflammatory disease! Choose whole food with no thickeners, gums, or mixing agents.
- **Choose organic** – organic foods are less likely to contain herbicides and pesticides that wreak havoc on your Microbiome, neurotransmitters, and hormone metabolism (more on those later in this chapter).
- **Filter drinking water** – chlorine and fluoride damage your gut mucous lining.

- **Avoid or minimize wheat and grains** – "We know with confidence given scientific research that the gliadin protein of wheat and related proteins of other grains increase intestinal permeability so that undigested food components, microbes and toxic breakdown products seep into the blood stream."[11] Ah, this isn't just me suggesting this . . . this is real science!
- **Reduce or eliminate alcohol** – alcohol and sugars can increase fungal overgrowth.
- **Get off NSAIDs or Non-Steroidal Anti-inflammatory drugs** (i.e. Ibuprofen),[12,13] and **stomach acid-suppressing drugs** (i.e. Omeprazole or Prilosec),[14] These drugs are known to cause gastropathy and enteropathy. In other words, your gut will *not* be happy, and you will be symptomatic sooner or later, if not sooner.

Let me bring this down to a personal level. In my mid-thirties, I slipped on some ice and fell down a small set of stairs (six steps) on my butt. As a result, I herniated C7-T1. The resultant pain in my right shoulder was day in and day out for years! I had chiropractic therapy two times a week, but nothing was helping. I had massages and on and on, and that didn't help either. So, what does a professional woman do who must get up and go to work each day? She wears an ice pack under her lab coat and takes ibuprofen, too. Daily. I had no idea that ibuprofen could damage my gut lining so badly.

As cited above ibuprofen can most definitely cause problems in the gut. Combine that with a gluten and dairy allergy, and you can get a wicked case of leaky gut syndrome. Once I made the dietary changes and did the other remedies to heal my gut,

I no longer had the pain or bloating associated with leaky gut syndrome.

Now that I've discussed some basics of improving your gut microbiome, I want to get very specific about a group of microbes in your gut that impact your hormone health—namely your estrobolome.

## The estrobolome

Most women and medical providers understand that estrogen is produced in the ovaries and the adrenals. However, the gut plays a very critical role in the regulation and reabsorption of estrogens—both healthy and toxic ones.

After entering your intestines, estrogen undergoes either elimination or reabsorption, circulating throughout your body to maintain an optimal balance essential for your well-being. Remarkably, this process is orchestrated by a "multidimensional set of processes" called your estrobolome bacteria.[15]

The estrobolome works by secreting an enzyme called beta-glucuronidase, which converts estrogen into its active forms. Again, these estrogens are then either expelled from the body or reabsorbed into circulation to carry out their functions. If toxic estrogens are reabsorbed, symptoms of estrogen dominance increase as does the risk of hormone related cancers—such as breast, ovarian, and prostate. That is why ensuring a healthy estrobolome is critical to prevent disease and ensure long-term vitality and longevity. (I'll discuss more on this below.)

However, here's the catch: the proper function of your estrobolome relies heavily on the health and diversity of microorganisms within your microbiome. Unfortunately, when the estrobolome encounters issues—a common occurrence affecting approximately 90 percent of people who report disruptive digestive symptoms—it not only disrupts digestion but also interferes with the delicate estrogen balance in your body.

Here's another interesting connection between estrogen and your gut—maintaining healthy estrogen levels supports optimal gut function by preserving the integrity of the gut lining and preventing leaky gut, creating a fabulous win-win relationship. The take home message, take care of your gut and your estrogen balance, and it will take care of you!

## Eating for your estrobolome

There is a common theme running throughout this book about eating a healthy, raw, organic diet filled with lots of vegetables, fruits, healthy fats, and clean protein. You now know that your diet choices significantly influence the composition of the estrobolome, with several dietary factors potentially benefiting its balance.

- Integrate cruciferous vegetables like broccoli, cauliflower, cabbage, and kale into your diet to regulate beneficial gut bacteria, supply fiber for gut health, and aid in the healthy detoxification of hormones, including estrogen.
- Opt for plant-based foods high in dietary fiber, such as nuts, seeds, legumes, beans, and a variety of vegetables, to support a healthy gut microbiota and achieve balanced estrogen levels. Notably, avocado and grapefruit showed promising effects in a study.
- Consume prebiotic foods rich in fructo-oligosaccharides or inulin, promoting the growth of beneficial bacteria. Options include chicory, asparagus, garlic, and banana.
- Incorporate fermented foods like sauerkraut, kimchi, and kvass to help restore gut bacteria and enhance diversity.

- Include probiotic strains such as Lactobacillus acidophilus to reduce the presence of bacteria producing beta-glucuronidase.

## Supplement if needed

When I see DUTCH (Dried Urine Testing for Comprehensive Hormones) test results for my clients, I can see how healthy their Phase 1 and Phase 2 liver metabolism is. I can also see Indican levels, which are often associated with gut dysbiosis (gut flora or bugs are out of balance). If—*after* implementing the recommended dietary changes above and eliminating toxic estrogens from their environment, food, and personal care products—the client still has high levels of toxic estrogens, then supplementation is the next step. One of my favorite and most effective supplements to add is Calcium-D-Glucarate, which steps in like a superhero and stops beta-glucuronidase in its tracks. This means that the toxic estrogens get shuttled out of the digestive track for good! See the Resources section for more information.

# Balance Your Nervous System

I'm sure you've heard of the distinctions "fight, flight, or freeze" when it comes to our nervous system. That reference describes our **S**ympathetic **N**ervous **S**ystem (SNS), what I like to call our **S**urvival **N**ervous **S**ystem. Our **P**ara**S**ympathetic **N**ervous **S**ystem (PSNS)—which I call our "**P**retty **S**afe **N**ervous **S**ystem"—is often referred to as the "rest and digest" nervous system. Whatever you want to call these two systems, they need to be balanced!

Our bodies are designed to handle stress, and some stress can be beneficial. But prolonged stress or SNS activity will result in chronic inflammation and destabilized natural repair processes, impacting cortisol, insulin, and glucose levels, which can all cause weight gain and diabetes. In her seminal book, *You Can Beat The Odds*,[16] Brenda Stockdale reminds us that "unrelenting stress is the incendiary spark that fuels the fires of internal destruction."

Indeed, our nervous system must have balance for us to live a long healthy life. Let's use an automobile analogy —if we had no way to cool the engine of our cars, our engines overheat and basically blow up! We need to remember that the SNS system must be "cooled" or *balanced* by the PSNS system to prevent the "internal destruction" that is highlighted in over 24,000 published medical articles.[17]

Researchers from Yale University School of Medicine found that meditating three times a week for six weeks improved endothelial function (the lining of our vessels from head to toe) and reduced blood pressure, resting heart rate, and the risk of heart disease.[18]

Let's face it, life has stress! However, stress in and of itself is not all bad. How we deal with it and how long the stress lasts are key factors in determining how stress effects the body. Stress can create some nasty biochemistry that can take a big toll on your body. Or, you can create new patterns with stress that can totally change the nasty negative biochemistry to healthy, happy, soothing biochemistry that supports your body.

Simple techniques like deep breathing, going for a walk, taking a short "Napitation," Meditation, Yoga, or other Yin-type exercises can help lower the stress and SNS force on the body. Using simple essential oils can help. For example, lavender and other oils are soothing. Lime and cilantro mixed in the palm of your hand, then rubbed down the side of your neck under the ears (on the Vagus nerve) can very quickly increase your PSNS. I use this technique every day and have tracked the quick and

significant response by using HRV (heart rate variability) tracking. It really works!

## Balance Your Neurotransmitters

Now that I've talked about gut health and its link to a plethora
of dis-ease states, including depression and anxiety, let's discuss
neurotransmitters and the gut–brain axis.

As stated above, the gut and brain are connected both biochemically and physically in various ways. The Vagus nerve, the
longest nerve in the body, goes from the brain to the gut and sends
signals in both directions. For instance, stress can send a message through the Vagus nerve and cause gastrointestinal (GI)
problems. Neurotransmitters like serotonin, dopamine, and
GABA are biochemical communicators that impact our feelings
and emotions. While serotonin is produced in the brain, a large
portion is also produced in the gut. Your gut microbiome also
produces Gamma-aminobutyric acid (or GABA for short). This
fabulous neurotransmitter can reduce anxiety and depression-
like behavior and is also amazing to calm restless leg syndrome
(RLS). Can you see the connection here? If you are eating foods
that disrupt your microbiome, then your risk of causing your
neurotransmitters to be out of whack is greatly increased.[19]

You may have some genetic variations (remember, Single
Nucleotide Polymorphisms or SNPs as discussed in Chapter 5),
that predispose you to some neurotransmitter imbalances such
as COMT, MAO, DRD 1 & 2, TH, and GAD-1. Variations in these
genes can have a profound impact on your mood, your executive
function, and even your sleep.[20] But even if you *do* have some
SNPs with your neurotransmitters, you do not have to be a victim to it. You may have to work harder to balance them, but you
still can be in charge of your mental health! Your diet and your

lifestyle will have a direct, dramatic impact. As mentioned in *Super Gut*, Dr. Davis clearly outlines habits that will support your gut. As you support your gut, you support your gut-brain axis.

You can support your gut-brain each day by eating clean, healthy, real food, avoiding sugar, and avoiding gluten, *or* you can have a bunch of junk food loaded with chemicals, preservatives, glyphosate, emulsifiers, and so on. You can choose if you fill your day to the brink with high-stress activities, or you can stop and take the time to breathe or meditate.

PubMed.gov—the online database of biomedical and lifestyle articles and abstracts—lists 354 citations about diaphragmatic breathing and stress. Really? Yes! If you broaden the search to just say breathing and stress, then over 18,000 citations pop up. There is no doubt that slow deep breathing (especially deep belly dia-phragmatic that I will discuss in detail in Chapter 18) will help balance your neurotransmitters and stress hormones. Deep breathing will activate your Vagus nerve, which turns on your ParaSympathetic Nervous system, and turns off the Sympathetic Nervous System.[21,22,23]

## Consider This

- Are there toxic substances in your home, your fridge, or your personal care products that might be sabotaging your estrobolome?

- What new foods can you add to support a healthy gut?

- What's a simple "floor" that you can add to your daily self-care to improve balance of your nervous system?

- What can you do on a daily basis to support a healthy microbiome?

*Fourteen*

# Balance Your Hormones

*"Hormones are the key to everything in women's health.
They are the foundation of our physical,
emotional and mental well-being."*
~ANNA CABECA, MD

Picture a symphony orchestra, with every musician playing their unique instrument to create a beautiful harmony. The conductor knows all of the parts and will bring all instrumentalists in on cue when it's time to perform their part. When the timing and pitch are perfect, the music is harmonious. When it's out of balance, cacophony can be created. Our bodies are like this; however, in our case, the master conductor is the endocrine system. When everything's working smoothly, you feel great. But when there's an imbalance, it's like a discordant note disrupting the melody of your health.

## Your Endocrine System

There are more than 200 hormones or hormone-like substances in the body; however, the ones most often in the spotlight are:

- Thyroid hormones
- Insulin
- Serotonin
- Progesterone

- Estrogens (estradiol, estriol, and estrone)
- Testosterone and/or Androgens
- Cortisol

The endocrine system is like a control center in your body that uses hormones as messengers to regulate various functions. Hormones are chemical substances produced by glands in different parts of your body, such as the thyroid, sex hormones, adrenal glands, pancreas, and more.

These hormones travel through your bloodstream to target organs and tissues, where they help regulate processes like metabolism, growth, reproduction, mood, and hunger. Think of hormones as little messenger molecules that tell your body what to do and when to do it.

For example, the thyroid gland produces hormones that control your metabolism, while the adrenal glands produce hormones that help you deal with stress. Meanwhile, the pancreas releases insulin to help regulate blood sugar levels.

Overall, the endocrine system plays a crucial role in keeping your body balanced and functioning properly, kind of like an internal communication network ensuring everything runs smoothly.

Water filters are a great analogy for what we need to do for our endocrine systems. If we do *not* filter or cleanse out the toxins, our entire endocrine system may get clogged up, just like dirty old water pipes.

Another way to look at our endocrine systems is by imagining a very old rusty padlock and key. On a cellular level, our cells respond like a lock and key system known as receptor sites. Many, many biochemical processes require this lock and key receptor system. If our receptor sites get clogged up with toxins (like a rusty old padlock) the key may not fit properly. In our body, that key may be a hormone or a biochemical cofactor/nutrient to make the hormones work. Often, the opposite can occur—the key may not be a healthy hormone or nutrient that our body needs, but a toxic ingredient that is a "hormone mimicker" or "endocrine disruptor." Either way, our receptor sites can get clogged with many inorganic waste products that block our cellular signals. Remember, I went into more depth on this in Chapter 11.

### Hormonal days and hormonal nights

For most women, when we talk of "hormonal days," we mean our sex hormones—estrogens, progesterone, and testosterone. Our "hormonal days" may include symptoms like PMS, morning sickness, unsightly acne, brain fog, bloating, hot flashes, insomnia, and mood swings—just to name a few!

Our sex hormones are responsible for regulating various bodily functions and processes, including menstruation, pregnancy, brain health, breast health, bone health, heart health, and menopause. When there is an imbalance in the hormones, it can lead to a variety of health issues.

For many of us, we miss the signals that our hormones are giving us (like those proverbial red dashboard lights in your car) and attempting to tell us that something is out of whack—until it becomes unbearable!

So, to increase your access to vitality, you must first be *aware*. Simply increasing your awareness of hormonal symptoms—the "dashboard lights"—will get you much closer to having an endocrine (hormone) system that is functioning optimally.

## Hormonal Imbalances

When your hormones are out of balance, everything seems to be much harder. It's harder to think, it's harder to get along, it's harder to be grounded and serene, not to mention having "spiritual poise," and it's certainly harder to avoid the temptation to eat fattening comfort foods and sweets. Your sex hormones impact nearly every area of your body. If your hormones are out of balance, then your body will *not* be functioning optimally. Period! (No pun intended.)

As an example, estrogen imbalance can impact the gut and alter the microbiome (as discussed in Chapter 13), which can cause bloating, constipation, discomfort, nausea, and diarrhea. The gut in turn creates the "estrobolome," which you now know is a microbiome solely dedicated to regulating estrogen. Additionally, estrogen/progesterone imbalances dramatically increase the risk of hormone-related cancers (think breasts, uterine, ovaries, and prostate). But it doesn't stop there—hormone imbalances impact brain function, hair and nail growth, and energy, and they cause visceral fat accumulation (fat around the belly), obesity, and poor libido. And that's just the impact of our sex hormones being out of whack! When you combine the above mess with chronic stress and the resulting elevated cortisol and blood sugar changes, things get even worse.

## Balance is Critical

To achieve hormonal harmony in your body, balance is critical. If you have ever watched a symphony perform, you know that there's a larger number of string instruments than there are woodwinds, brass, and percussion instruments to create the balance of sound needed for the piece to be beautifully balanced.

In a symphony orchestra, there are typically two flute players, one oboe, one clarinet, one bassoon, one or two trumpets, two French horns, one trombone, and a tuba. When I attended the Atlanta Symphony Orchestra to enjoy Mahler's huge 72-minute blockbuster 5th symphony, there were two additional flutes, two additional oboes, two additional clarinets, two additional bassoons, four additional horns, two additional trumpets, two additional trombones, then tuba, timpani, percussion, harp, and strings. The sound from the woodwinds and brass was enormous and amazing! Yet, if the rest of the orchestra included the normal number of string players, the sound would have been way out of balance and sounded terrible. To compensate for the big sound of the horns and to keep the beautiful symphonic sound balanced, the string section also had to be increased. For example, instead of the traditional six or seven cellos, for Mahler's 5th, three more cellos were added. Instead of four to six contrabasses (the big upright bass), four more were added.

Your hormones compensate for balance and harmony in a similar way.

Imagine your endocrine system (your hormonal factory, if you will) like a symphony, where various hormones play distinct roles that all need to be balanced for hormonal harmony. Like the symphony, if one hormone is out of balance or takes center stage, it can overshadow the other hormones and create a cacophony of symptoms instead of beautiful hormonal harmony. These messenger molecules are unable to deliver their proper message to specific hormone-related tissues, and thus you are left feeling upset, unwell, and off-balance.

## Yin and yang energy

I'm sure you are aware of the beautiful balance of yin and yang or feminine and masculine energies. When they are in balance, it's beautiful. When they are out of balance, they can create some significant challenges—even physically.

Men were divinely designed to protect, provide, produce results, day after day, procreate, and preside. As a result, to fuel them, they have at least sixteen times more testosterone than women do. The challenge in our modern world is that many women are trying to produce the same kind of results that men's bodies were designed to do. Whether we are running on fumes raising a young family, or climbing the professional ladder, or both, our bodies were not designed to produce these same long days, day in and day out. Unfortunately, that hasn't stopped us. In part it's because we have not been taught about these hormonal differences and what extended masculine or yang energy does to our hormone balance.

Again, men's results are fueled by testosterone. For women, with limited supply of testosterone, we quicky turn to cortisol to produce results. That's the rub or where the fallout begins.

This may not be a major problem if the stress is short term. But, in our modern world, the pattern for most is chronic, daily, unrelenting stress. As women, when we are dealing with deadlines or daily to-do lists, whether working women or stay at home moms, we are still producing results that need a lot of energy! Deadlines seem to turn on yang energy, which requires a lot more testosterone.

Can you begin to see the dilemma we face in the modern world? When we, as women, are working long hard hours, the cortisol demand is higher, thus the progesterone demand is higher.

### Stress and prolonged yang energy

I'm sure you've heard that stress causes a cascade of events that raises cortisol. When stress hits the **H**ypothalamus (an area of the brain), then it sends a signal to the **P**ituitary (another area of the brain), which signals the **A**drenal glands to produce cortisol. (Note—this is referred to as the **HPA** Axis. If you see this in the literature or online, now you know what they are referring to.)

Without getting too technical with hormonal biochemistry, I want to elucidate a few things about how stress causes hormonal imbalance and the subsequent health challenges.

Pregnenolone is a master hormone that converts biochemically to progesterone—the "life giving" hormone. Per the very simplified hormonal cascade diagram in Figure 1 below, you can see that progesterone converts down to cortisol and over to the androgens (male hormones) and estrogens. If cortisol is ramped up high (note the bold arrow) then progesterone can be depleted quickly. This phenomenon is known as "progesterone steal." The stress, and resultant cortisol spike is "stealing" or sucking dry the reserves of progesterone.

## SIMPLIFIED STEROID (SEX) HORMONE PATHWAY

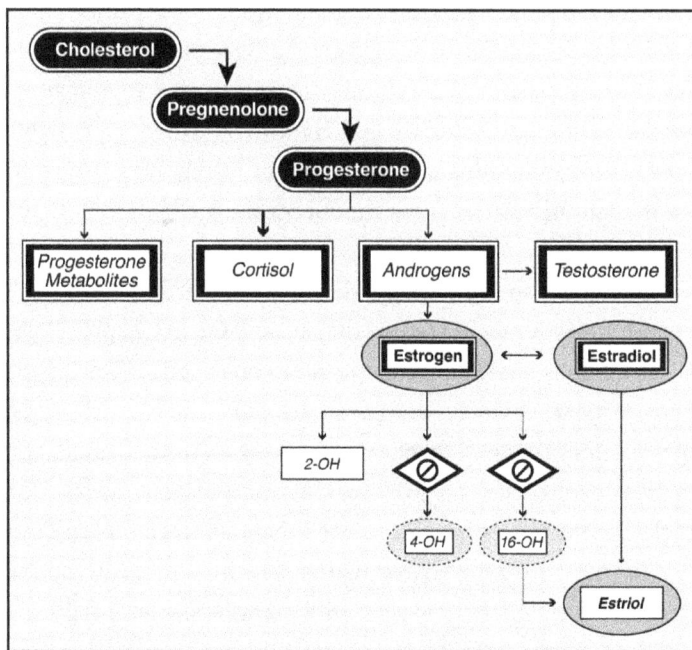

Figure 1: Note that Cortisol, with the bold arrow, has a significant impact on hormonal balance, especially for women.

## Estrogen Dominance

While both estrogen and progesterone play essential roles in the female body, they need to be balanced to function optimally.

When stress is high and progesterone is being used[1] on high demand, it creates an imbalance between progesterone (P) and estrogen (E), often referred to as the P:E ratio. If the relative progesterone (P) is lower than the estrogen (E), or if you have "progesterone deficiency" (as is the case with perimenopausal and menopausal women) then "estrogen dominance" can be present. Even if you have *normal* levels of progesterone but have an abundance of *fake* estrogens in your body (from numerous sources in our world today), then you also have estrogen dominance (see below).

To take this one step further, many women can't understand how they can have estrogen "dominance" when they are suffering from estrogen deficiency symptoms during the perimenopausal years (i.e., hot flashes and vaginal dryness). However, you can *still* have estrogen dominance *if* the amount of relative estrogen is more than the relative progesterone. Again, it comes back to the P:E *ratio*.

Now, I need to clean up a myth that goes back to the Women's Health Initiative (WHI) study that I discussed in Chapter 3. Not all estrogen is bad! Synthetic estrogens do *not* equal God-given, nature made, divinely designed estrogens. In fact, it's when our natural estrogen levels drop, during perimenopause and menopause, that our rates of breast cancer and heart disease skyrocket. Synthetic estrogens, on the other hand, can increase our risk of these diseases. To summarize, a drop in progesterone or progesterone deficiency—seen with excess stress and/or during perimenopause—can cause an excess of estrogen or "estrogen dominance."

## Causes of estrogen dominance

**Stress** – Again, as mentioned above, prolonged stress , with the resultant high cortisol levels depletes progesterone, creating a relative imbalance between progesterone and estrogen.

**Diet** – Consuming processed and high-fat foods and foods with pesticides, herbicides, food coloring, and nasty preservatives can increase estrogen levels in the body, as these substances are sources of fake or foreign, synthetic estrogens

**Iatrogenic (doctor caused)** – Birth control pills and/or synthetic hormone replacement therapy are additional examples of fake estrogens that will disrupt the healthy progesterone and estrogen balance.

**Xenoestrogens** – "Xeno" means foreign. These are the foreign, toxic, human-made estrogens that we are barraged with daily that will cause estrogen dominance.

Here's a list of common sources of xenoestrogens that you should try to avoid:

- **Skincare:**
  - 4-Methylbenzylidene camphor (4-MBC) (sunscreen lotions)
  - Parabens (methylparaben, ethylparaben, propyl-paraben and butylparaben commonly used as a preservative)
  - Benzophenone (sunscreen lotions)
- **Nail polish and nail polish remover**
- **Industrial products and plastics:**
  - Bisphenol A (monomer for polycarbonate plastic and epoxy resin; antioxidant in plasticizers)
  - Phthalates (plasticizers)
  - DEHP (plasticizer for PVC)

- Polybrominated biphenyl ethers (PBDEs) (flame retardants used in plastics, foams, building materials, electronics, furnishings, motor vehicles).
- Polychlorinated biphenyls (PCBs)

- **Food:**
  - Erythrosine / FD&C Red No. 3
  - Phenosulfothiazine (a red dye)
  - Butylated hydroxyanisole / BHA (food preservative)

- **Building supplies:**
  - Pentachlorophenol (general biocide and wood preservative)
  - Polychlorinated biphenyls / PCBs (in electrical oils, lubricants, adhesives, paints)

- **Insecticides:**
  - Atrazine (weed killer)
  - DDT (insecticide, banned)
  - Dichlorodiphenyldichloroethylene (one of the breakdown products of DDT)
  - Dieldrin (insecticide)
  - Endosulfan (insecticide)
  - Heptachlor (insecticide)
  - Lindane / hexachlorocyclohexane (insecticide, used to treat lice and scabies)
  - Methoxychlor (insecticide)
  - Fenthion
  - Nonylphenol and derivatives (industrial surfactants; emulsifiers for emulsion polymerization; laboratory detergents; pesticides)

- **Other:**
  - Propyl gallate
  - Chlorine and chlorine by-products

- Ethinylestradiol (combined oral contraceptive pill)
- Metalloestrogens (a class of inorganic xenoestrogens)
- Alkylphenol (surfactant used in cleaning detergents
- **Pesticides:**
  - Glyphosphate

Here's a guide to minimize your personal exposure to xenoestrogens:

**Food**

- Avoid all pesticides, herbicides, and fungicides.
- Choose organic, locally grown and in-season foods.
- Peel non-organic fruits and vegetables.
- Buy hormone-free meats and dairy products to avoid hormones and pesticides.

**Plastics**

- Reduce the use of plastics whenever possible.
- Do not microwave food in plastic containers.
- Avoid the use of plastic wrap to cover food for storing or microwaving.
- Use glass or ceramics whenever possible to store food.
- Do not leave plastic containers, especially your drinking water, in the sun.
- If a plastic water container has heated up significantly, throw it away.
- Don't refill plastic water bottles.
- Avoid freezing water in plastic bottles to drink later.

**Household Products**

- Use chemical free, biodegradable laundry and household cleaning products.

- Choose chlorine-free products and unbleached paper products (i.e., tampons, menstrual pads, toilet paper, paper towel, coffee filters).
- Use a chlorine filter on shower heads and filter drinking water.

**Health and Beauty Products**

- Avoid creams and cosmetics that have toxic chemicals and estrogenic ingredients such as parabens and stearalkonium chloride.
- Minimize your exposure to nail polish and nail polish removers.
- Use naturally based fragrances, such as essential oils.
- Use chemical free soaps and toothpastes.
- Read the labels on condoms and diaphragm gels.

**At the Office**

- Be aware of noxious gas such as from copiers and printers, carpets, fiberboards, and at the gas pump.

If you want to learn more, check out the Resources section.

Source: womeninbalance.org

## Symptoms of estrogen dominance

There are several symptoms of estrogen dominance, and you don't need to have all of them to qualify for it. Additionally, you may have some of these symptoms *screaming* at you (like an 8, 9, or 10 on a 1 to 10 scale) and others that are barely noticeable.

Are you experiencing any of these?

- Anxiety
- Abdominal pain and bloating
- Brain fog

- Breast tenderness
- Constipation
- Cyclical acne
- Depression
- Endometriosis
- Extreme hunger and cravings
- Fatigue
- Fibroids (breast or uterine)
- Hair loss
- Headaches
- Heavy or excessive bleeding
- Insomnia
- Irregular menstrual periods
- Low libido
- Mood swings
- PMS/PMDD
- Poor memory
- Water retention
- Weight gain (especially around the middle)

Although the above symptoms are aggravating and may decrease your quality of life, the most serious consequence of estrogen dominance is an increased risk of breast cancer. Estrogen dominance (again, often synonymous with progesterone deficiency) causes many physical and emotional problems at midlife. On an average, as women go through the perimenopausal years, estrogen may fall 30 to 50 percent. Progesterone, on the other hand, has been said by some experts to drop as low as 100 percent! Can you see how the estrogen dominance scenario gets worse at midlife?

Several studies have found that insufficient progesterone may be a more important factor than excessive estrogen in increasing a woman's risk of breast cancer.[2,3] One of the most significant studies of the relationship between low levels of natural progesterone and increased breast cancer risk was published in the *American Journal of Epidemiology* in August 1981.[4] In this study, conducted by researchers from Johns Hopkins University's School of Public Health, women of childbearing age who were having difficulty conceiving were divided into two groups.

The first group consisted of women whose infertility was attributed to progesterone deficiency, while the second group was composed of women with infertility due to nonhormonal causes. All the women were followed for thirteen to thirty-three years, and the incidence of breast cancer in each group was recorded.

At the study's conclusion, researchers found that the infertile women with progesterone deficiency had a premenopausal breast cancer risk that was 540 times greater than that of women whose infertility was not related to their hormone status. Not only that, but these women also had a 1,000 times greater risk of death from all types of cancer. After menopause, when estrogen levels declined, the breast cancer risk was similar in the two groups, suggesting that progesterone's protective effects were much more critical during the premenopausal period.

An interesting thing to consider is that, with these kinds of results in a clinical trial dating back to 1981, why wasn't this published all over and shouted from the rooftops? Why have women *not* been told about this important message?

## Restore Your Hormonal Balance

Estrogen dominance is a big deal and needs to be managed to regain hormonal balance.

Below are some tips to support you in optimizing your hormonal balance.

## Manage your stress

Practice deep breathing exercises

I have software on my computers that will gray out the screen every fifteen minutes, for fifteen seconds, to protect my eyes from eye strain and blue light. I have found it very helpful to "habit stack" and use this screen saving time to take slow deep abdominal breaths every fifteen to thirty minutes. Try it.

Monitor your heart rate variability (HRV)

This will help to increase your awareness of your stress levels in real time. Elite HRV is one app that trains you with biofeedback that can help you to: improve your breathing, enhance your calm states to decrease your Sympathetic Nervous System (SNS) response, increase your Parasympathetic (PSNS) Nervous System response, and raise your HRV score. The OURA ring is another great option to monitor your HRV. However, I make sure that I keep the Bluetooth turned off when I'm wearing it. The last thing you need is that constant exposure to EMF when you're trying to track your health. I take mine off, turn the Bluetooth on, get my results, then turn off the Bluetooth before I wear it again. It's that smart. It will track your data regardless of the Bluetooth capacity. WOW, technology can be so cool. And, yes, so risky, too.

Enjoy lime and clove essential oils

Put one drop of each oil in the palm of your hand. Combine them (rub them in a clockwise position to blend them), and then rub the combined oils down both sides of your neck under your ear, along your Vagus nerve. This will also decrease your SNS (stress nervous system) and increase your PSNS (pretty safe nervous system). See the Resources section.

Practice yoga

Because yoga is so instrumental in supporting breath work, which in turn increases PSNS activity, it's a very effective way to decrease your cortisol levels.

Use CBD oil

Joy Organics is the brand I recommend to my clients. They have the highest ranking in the industry.

## Avoid toxins

Examine your fridge, your pantry, and your yard care to find hidden sources of toxins as part of your environmental cleanse (discussed in Chapter 9). Start with switching out one toxic food and replacing it with a live, healthy organic choice.

The Environmental Working Group (EWG)[5] is an excellent resource to check all products you are exposed to and see the toxic load they may contain. EWG also has incredible resources to choose healthier products. Refer to the "Dirty Dozen" and "Clean Fifteen" for a place to start.[6]

Skin Deep is a subsidiary of EWG. They have an enormous database of personal care products so you can assess the toxic load of your products when deciding what's best for your body and skin.

Start with one product at a time. If you are unable to toss all of your toxic products at once due to cost, then at least replace each new product with a "clean" or "green product" after your old toxic product runs out.

## Increase your greens

By now you know how I feel about consuming healthy greens! The steroid (sex hormone) pathway has over 45 biochemical conversions from cholesterol, to pregnenolone, to progesterone, to all other hormones. Every single step in that process requires good healthy water and *greens*. I know I've said it before but be sure to increase your greens and veggies—especially cruciferous veggies like cabbage, kale, broccoli, brussel sprouts and even cauliflower.

## Replenishing your hormones as you age

Now that I have discussed estrogen dominance, I want to clarify and reinforce that estrogen is *vital* to your health! The estrogens that God designed our bodies to make is vital. It's the toxic man-made estrogens above that are what we have to be careful of.

Many women are scared to death of estrogen, as the media and their doctors have told them, "It causes breast cancer." Why on earth would God give everyone estrogen if it causes breast cancer? In fact, Dr. Jennifer Simmons, renowned former breast cancer surgeon in Philadelphia, now specializing in Functional Medicine, has said, "To say that estrogen causes breast cancer is absurd … When your body can't access its own estrogen because the ovaries are shutting down, breast cancer becomes an issue!"[7] Ladies, that is another reason why breast cancer is prevalent in menopausal women.

One other point that Dr. Simmons makes about the story of estrogen causing breast cancer is because of Big Pharma. We have drugs that block estrogen synthesis and act on the estrogen receptors. She states, "so the explanation of estrogen causing breast cancer is for the purpose of utilizing these drugs, NOT because estrogen causes breast cancer."[8] There you have it!

## The benefits of bioidentical hormone replacement therapy

Chemically identical to hormones produced by the body, bioidentical hormones (BHRT) are derived from plant estrogens and come in a variety of forms including pills, gels, suppositories, and injections that allow for ease of use and increase treatment adherence. BHRT is often prescribed as patients age and their hormone levels begin to decrease, especially in the case of women who enter perimenopause or menopause to improve the moderate-to-severe symptoms associated with this transition. Furthermore, hormone replacement therapies have been found to reduce the risk for diabetes, tooth loss, and cataracts while potentially improving skin thickness, hydration, and elasticity. For post-treatment cancer patients with decreased estrogen levels, BHRT has shown efficacy in improving general well-being and overall quality of life; it may also alleviate some treatment-related symptoms such as migraines and insomnia.

## Compounded bioidentical hormones and FDA regulation

Custom made by pharmacies per physicians' orders, compounded bioidentical hormones typically include ingredients combined or altered to meet the specific needs of an individual patient. While such formulations may be effective when tailored correctly, it is important to note that the FDA has not approved any custom-compounded bioidentical hormone therapies to date. As such, clinicians are encouraged to maintain caution in prescribing compounded bioidentical hormones.

The hormonal specialists that study with the American College of Anti-Aging Medicine (A4M) receive specific courses on bioidentical hormones and teaching physicians how critically important bioidentical hormones are. These specialists basically say, "Look, we wear glasses and hearing aids because our body is aging, and we're not afraid to support them. Why is it that we think that we can't support our health with bioidentical hormones?" We give thyroid support, but we can't support our sex hormones? That's crazy to me.

Like your skeleton, your bioidentical hormones will support you.[9]

## Optimize Your Hormone Metabolism

Hormone metabolism is unfortunately not talked about or measured regularly in Western medicine. However, this aspect of hormonal health is every bit as important as your overall hormone levels—especially when it comes to estrogen.

Most women have heard of the BRCA gene mutation that can increase one's risk of breast cancer; however, there is considerable misunderstanding about this gene. Every human has both the BRCA1 and BRCA2 genes. Despite what their names might suggest, BRCA genes do not cause breast cancer. On the contrary, these genes normally play a big role in *preventing* breast cancer. BRCA genes are actually known as tumor suppressor genes because they help *repair* DNA *breaks* that can lead to cancer and the uncontrolled growth of tumors.[10]

Perhaps you've heard women say "I have the BRCA gene" or "I do not have the BRCA gene" when they are discussing their risk of developing breast cancer. Here's the deal—unless your BRCA gene is NULL, we all have the BRCA gene. The BRCA gene is actually the BReast CAncer gene. Its function is to actually spot breast cancer and eliminate it ASAP. If you "have" the BRCA gene, it typically means that you have an alteration, variation, or mutation in this gene, and it may be functioning at only 60 percent or even 30 percent of its capacity. Thus, the DNA repair is not happening as it should be.

You can see in Figure 2,[11] in the far-left corner, a little box that says BRCA1 and BRCA2. Note that this genetic mutation is only one tiny sliver of the causes of breast cancer. See the outer list on the right with plant estrogens all the way down to food additives—these are the nasty xenoestrogens that we are bombarded with every day. This is the vital information you have not been getting from conventional dysfunctional medicine. These xenoestrogens change the expression of your DNA and can actually cause all hormone-related cancers, including prostate cancer. These are the substances that you can eliminate from your diet, your personal care, your yard care, etc.[12]

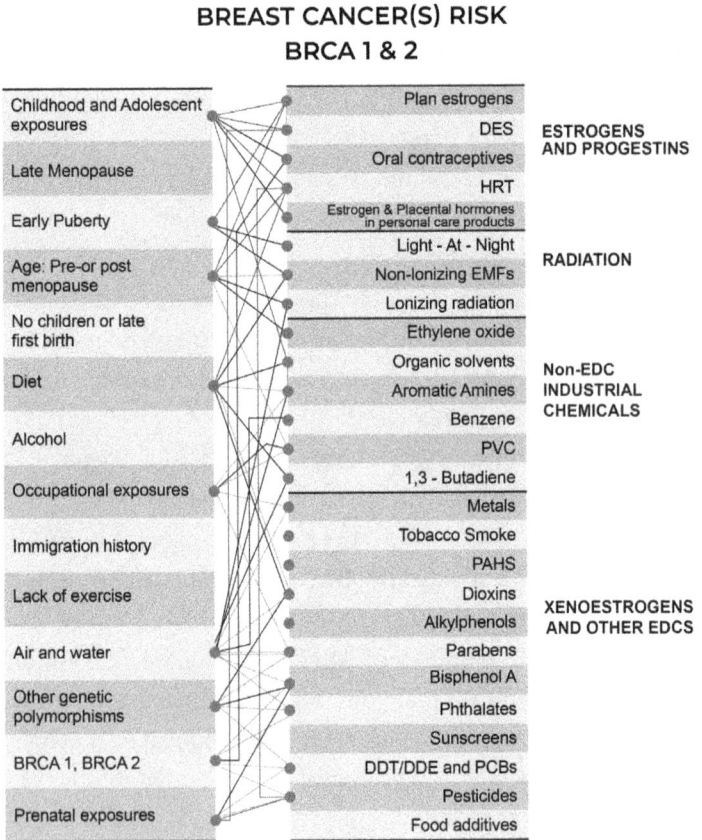

## BREAST CANCER(S) RISK
## BRCA 1 & 2

| | |
|---|---|
| Childhood and Adolescent exposures | Plan estrogens |
| | DES |
| Late Menopause | Oral contraceptives |
| | HRT |
| Early Puberty | Estrogen & Placental hormones in personal care products |
| | Light - At - Night |
| Age: Pre-or post menopause | Non-Ionizing EMFs |
| | Ionizing radiation |
| No children or late first birth | Ethylene oxide |
| | Organic solvents |
| Diet | Aromatic Amines |
| | Benzene |
| Alcohol | PVC |
| | 1,3 - Butadiene |
| Occupational exposures | Metals |
| | Tobacco Smoke |
| Immigration history | PAHS |
| | Dioxins |
| Lack of exercise | Alkylphenols |
| | Parabens |
| Air and water | Bisphenol A |
| | Phthalates |
| Other genetic polymorphisms | Sunscreens |
| BRCA 1, BRCA 2 | DDT/DDE and PCBs |
| | Pesticides |
| Prenatal exposures | Food additives |

ESTROGENS AND PROGESTINS

RADIATION

Non-EDC INDUSTRIAL CHEMICALS

XENOESTROGENS AND OTHER EDCS

Figure 2: Complexity of Breast Cancer Causation
*Note: Lines indicate some of the many links*

You can test for the BRCA gene; however, I would rather my clients focus on the genes that they can *do* something about and have a profound impact on, each day. These genes are the genes that support hormone metabolism.

I want to again share this simplified hormone biochemistry cascade graphic in which you can see the three types of estrogen—estrone, estradiol, and estriol (refer to Figure 1 on Page 155). You will also see in these images that there are three chemical compounds: 2-OH, 4-OH, and 16-OH. The "OH" stands for hydroxylation. This is all part of what we call "phase one liver metabolism." Healthy phase one metabolism of estrogens *reduces* your risk of hormone-related cancers. Whereas the unhealthy phase one metabolism *increases* the risk.

Bear with me as I share some technical DNA information. I am doing so because it's easy to track with a DUTCH test, and there are simple steps to improve the function and thereby reduce your risk of cancers.

Two hydroxylation (2-OH) is considered healthy and is directly affected by the CYP1A1 gene. Sixteen hydroxylation (16-OH) is unhealthy and is impacted by the CYP34A gene. The CYP1B1 gene is what impacts 4 hydroxylation (4- OH), the most dangerous, as it can directly damage DNA by the formation of reactive oxygen species and other mechanisms.[13]

Let me share a client story to illustrate my point.

A 33-year-old women, mother of seven, approached me with continuing symptoms of severe abdominal cramping during her cycle. Eighteen months earlier she had undergone hysterectomy for endometriosis. So, her Western-trained Ob-Gyn took out her *part*, but did NOT address the root cause—her toxic burden or xenoestrogens that were causing her estrogen dominance and severe symptoms. Taking out her "part" did not relieve her symptoms long term. The initial endometriosis was eliminated with the removal of her uterus, but, as is often the case, endometriosis can spread outside of the uterus. Thus, because the "root cause" (poor hormone balance and poor hormone metabolism) that was creating the *dysfunction* was not addressed, the endometriosis and subsequent symptoms returned. Addressing cleansing of the toxins and supporting cellular function was what was needed.

When I see the pattern of high 16-OH or 4-OH metabolism with clients, I recommend Glutathione support and a lot of cruciferous veggies (as I do for most issues discussed in this book), resveratrol, and other supplements to help support this Phase 1 liver metabolism. Anything you can do to enhance liver health will support healthy hormone metabolism. Take a look at the list in Chapter 8 for tips on cleansing and supporting your liver.

## Monitoring your hormone levels and hormone metabolism

Early on in my career of working with hormones, I would have to use urine, blood, and saliva tests to get a better picture or what was going on with any client. Blood levels alone were just not enough. Today however, I'm thrilled to be able to use the DUTCH test—the most comprehensive hormone test on the market. The "Dried Urine Testing for Comprehensive Hormones" (DUTCH) analysis provides more detailed information about hormone levels than traditional blood tests. It not only measures your hormones, but shows the big picture of hormone metabolism. Additionally, you will get a detailed picture of your adrenal glands and can see clearly how your cortisol may be impacting your hormonal balance. Still other measures, like the "Organic Acids Test," reveal information about gut health, levels of inflammation, and even neurotransmitters.

Dr. Tara Scott, a nationally recognized authority on hormones and wellness, reiterated what I have been telling clients for some time:

*"The Standard of Care (what is considered the normal recommendations by western medicine) should be that women should get the DUTCH test at ages 25, 35, 45, 55."*

Hormonal harmony, balance, and metabolism are all critical to optimizing your DNA and your own personal vitality! (See the Resources section for $100 off the DUTCH test.)

## Consider This

- What is one floor that you could implement today to improve your hormonal harmony?

- Can you see certain toxins that you can begin to reduce or eliminate that would optimize your hormone balance?

- What are some ways that you can reduce your stress load to support optimal hormone balance?

# Section 7

## Divine Embodiment

## *Fifteen*

# Whole Body Alignment

*"Being a Queen starts right there—with being.*
*So if we're constantly doing, doing, doing there isn't any space –*
*mental, emotional or time space—to just be, let alone be our very*
*best qualities. And, there is the problem of embodiment …*
*to be our best qualities, we first have to,*
*literally, get those qualities in our bodies."*
~ALISON ARMSTRONG

E mbodiment encompasses various facets: To give tangible
form to abstract concepts, to exemplify ideas through action,
to unify disparate elements into a cohesive whole, to embrace
our existence. Embodiment is the expression of the Creation
Principles described in Chapter 6.

Remember that vitality is only created when we combine our
spiritual, emotional, mental, and physical bodies into our vision
for our Future-Self. All four must be aligned and integrated in
order for embodiment to occur.

Are you being a conscious creator of whole-body alignment?

You are creating daily through what you see, say, think, feel,
and do. You can use your creative powers to uplift, grow, change,
and spiral up through spiritual creation, or you can use these
powers to spiral downward on each level—spiritually, emotionally, mentally, and physically.

Remember, when we combine each of these levels with *spiritual creation* it looks like this:

Spiritual – to SEE

Mental – to SAY, including what we say to ourselves, as well as what we THINK on a subconscious level

Emotional – to FEEL

Physical – to DO

If you are unhealthy or out of balance in any one of your four bodies, you cannot achieve vitality. You are, in actuality, disembodied.

# On Being Disembodied

In our modern, hectic, fast-paced world, many of us go through life *disembodied*. In other words, our spiritual, emotional, mental, and physical bodies are not in sync. Perhaps this habit came from our needs being ignored, invalidated, or gaslit. Even worse, perhaps we became disembodied because of trauma or abuse. For some, we drive our bodies through task after task to avoid dealing with emotional heartache. Others may be stuck in their heads and completely ignore their bodies. Thus, the dangers of disembodiment can be that we are less sensitive to our body's signals, which can definitely pose a significant health risk. Another danger of disembodiment or dissociation from our body is that it may silence or exclude us from the deep ways of knowing, as Dr. Bessel van der Kolk so aptly taught in *The Body Keeps the Score*.[1] However, if we are dissociated or disembodied, then we may be deaf to the toll that is mounting.

Disembodied practices are as connected to your vitality as embodied ones. If your thoughts and emotions are low, your motivation follows. If you select dead food (also known as the Standard American Diet of highly processed, not-living food), you're actively sabotaging your gut's microbiome and, as a result, your mood and brain function as well. Lalah Delia, author of *Vibrate Higher Daily*, holds that the journey to a higher vibration begins with high vibrational, organic, raw, healthy foods.[2]

I understand this disembodiment all too well. I was clueless about my own degree of disembodiment for years. One of the driving forces for creating this book was to help teach those younger than I how to listen to and heal all parts to create true vitality.

## Have Reverence

Embodiment begins with having reverence for our bodies. The scriptures identify our bodies as temples:

> Know ye not that ye are the temple of God,
> and that the Spirit of God dwelleth in you?
> If any man defile the temple of God, him shall God destroy;
> for the temple of God is holy, which temple ye are.[3]

God commands us to have reverence for our body. We enhance that respect when we honor the connection of our spiritual, emotional, mental, and physical bodies.

## Being and Doing to Become Your Future-Self

Embodiment requires both *being* and *doing*. I have personally and professionally experienced the infinitely looped connection between these. *Being* refers to your thoughts, beliefs, and emotions. *Doing* is all about the actions you take. If you use the infinity symbol, think of the being on one side and the doing on the other, with the mid-point being embodiment.

When your thoughts, beliefs, and emotions are aligned, then your *being* inspires aligned actions. On the other hand, when taking action brings balance to the physical body, that *doing* can inspire the foundation for balanced moods, thoughts, and feelings.

The art and practice of embodied vitality can be achieved as outlined in the chapters ahead. Whether you begin with your *being* or *doing*, the pair are interconnected. For some, the *doing* aspect requires primary attention just to gain some footing for *being*. Others feel more empowered by first *being*. For the purpose of aligning with Creation Principles, I will first discuss the *being* side of this harmonic balance—the spiritual, mental, and emotional bodies—in Chapters 16 and 17. The *doing* side of this harmonic balance will be discussed in Chapter 18, where you can learn how to practice the Daily Vitals to enhance your physical body.

For your best experience, lean in and seek divine guidance and your intuition, to find *your* best personal place to embody your Future-Self to Create the Vitality You Crave.

## Consider This

- What would your Future-Self do if she were physically fit?

- What would you eat today if you cared about your physiology?

- What would you do to anchor your Future-Self in reality?

*Sixteen*

# Create Your Calm from Within

> *"Stress is an alarm clock that lets you know you're
> attached to something that is not true for you."*
>
> ~BYRON KATIE

A s our world continues to evolve (I get that is debatable), the stressors—spiritual, emotional, mental and physical, have evolved as well. Depression and suicide are on the rise. Our children are struggling with their identity. Our rates of disease continue to soar. These are all stressors that we have created. We can now choose to mitigate the stress and therefore the impact on our *being* with some simple practices.

In my own quest to restore my vitality, I discovered that, until I was able to learn the art of letting go, meditation, and being grateful for the abundance all around me, stress continued to knock on a daily basis. In this chapter I will address the incredible toll of stress and the tools I've learned to create my ability to be serene instead of stressed out.

## Understand the Science of Stress

There is significant science on the role of stress and dis-ease. More than 345,000 articles are cited in PubMed as of April 2024. As discussed in Chapter 14, stress sends signals to the **H**ypothalamus of the brain, which then signals the **P**ituitary, and then the

Adrenals—known as the HPA axis. When this cascade is enacted, it increases cortisol production, which will then begin a cascade of hormonal imbalance, insulin/glucose imbalance, and cardiovascular results (blood pressure, heart rate). It also impacts the endothelium (the inner lining of the heart and all of the vessels).

Internationally renowned Neuroscientist and Pharmacologist Candace Pert, PhD, author of *Molecules of Emotion*,[1] showed that our immune system is impacted by our emotions. Her research revealed that each "door-lock" on your white blood cells is precisely designed to receive a specific "key" or neuropeptide from the emotion centers of the brain. Dr. Pert was the pioneer of the Body-Mind medicine field and is one of the greatest experts of the 20th century. Her research revealed that every single nerve in our body and brain is modulated by messenger molecules. These messenger molecules create a communication that connects our mind, emotions, and behavior.

In the Journal of Neurology,[2] an eight-year study with 20,000 participants, revealed that the risk of stroke was more related to psychological distress than to cigarette smoking, blood pressure, obesity, heart attack history, diabetes, family history, stroke, or cholesterol level.

A Finnish study[3] evaluated more than 10,000 women over fifteen years and examined the relationship between stress and breast cancer. The study said, "Our data suggest that (stressful) life events increase breast cancer risk independently of body mass index, weight change, alcohol use, smoking and physical inactivity …" Researchers are not saying that stress *causes* cancer, but the mechanisms are clear: stress can modify how the immune system works and increase the risk of our being vulnerable to disease.

Other fascinating information in the field of mind/body medicine and stress has been cited by Dr. Barry Bittman, neurologist and medical director from Meadville Medical Center.[4] His research shows that we each have our own unique molecular response to stress that he has dubbed our "stress signature." His research, and that of others, reveals that once the genes are turned on due to stress, they can then also be turned off by implementing healthy strategies.

These research results and citations discussed above are just the very tip of the iceberg of proof that stress can impact the expression of our DNA as well as our chances of getting dis-ease or, at a minimum, feeling unwell and off-balance. You can do simple things to decrease your stress, like taking a deep breath. Breath is an essential part of your Daily Vitals as we will discuss in Chapter 18, and it is *the single most important skill* for calming your body and mind. In *You Can Beat the Odds*,[5] renowned Psychoneuroimmunologist Brenda Stockdale, MS, says: "Proper breathing is the royal road to calming you down and returning your body to balance." Breathing can help you shift from running on what I call the "Survival Nervous System" (SNS), but you could just as easily call it your "Stressed-out Nervous System."

## Understand Diffuse Awareness

We as women have "Diffuse Awareness." Diffuse means pouring out in every direction. That is precisely where our attention goes—in every direction. We as women have been genetically designed to be able to pay attention to more than one thing at a time. This of course can be a great blessing.

We can cook a multi-course meal and have it all arrive to the table just perfectly timed. We can watch the children out of the corner of our eye while we are cooking up that masterpiece. If we're professional women, we can do this at work as well. In my critical care nursing days, I could keep multiple monitors in my eyesight, while noticing every detail of my patient. At the same time, I could hear when another nurse called for sudden help. If you're in a professional office, I imagine you can be working on one task, overhearing conversations next to you, and noticing if your boss walks in the room.

Unfortunately, there is also a downside to our "Diffuse Awareness." We notice everything! Have you ever walked into a room and noticed a picture hanging crooked? It's like the picture is screaming at us, "fix me, I'm crooked!" We walk into a room with one intention, and then see something out of place, and then get sidetracked handling that instead. It's crazy, but women do it all the time. And it can leave us absolutely exhausted! There will *always* be something to do and something that is calling for our attention.

Diffuse awareness keeps us "on" all the time. Being "on" all the time is a significant silent stressor. This is why I recommend that women create Zone Time and Margin to increase the amount of time we are "off."

## Create Zone Time

Have you noticed that sometimes you can become swept away and time just slips by? You may have experienced being so single-focused on reading a great book that sixty minutes goes by in what seems like sixty seconds. Zone time for women is, amazingly, the only time we *effortlessly* get single-focused and when the noise quiets down.

"*Zone Time*" for you may be:
- Reading a good book
- Watching a good flick
- Talking with a girlfriend
- Gardening
- Dancing

- Playing an instrument
- Listening to music
- Walking in your neighborhood

To find the Zone Time that's right for you, start noticing which activities just sweep you away. Spend at least a few minutes each day doing one of these activities, and you'll find that it actually can help fill your vitality tank!

## Create Margin

In his landmark book, MARGIN (2004),[6] Dr. Richard Swenson, MD, wrote about the epidemic we are all experiencing of overwhelmed and overloaded lives. In his years of clinical practice as an internist, he concluded that much of the illness he diagnosed was from overloaded lives—on every level. Due to our contemporary stressors of change, mobility, expectations, time pressure, work, control, fear, relationships, competition, and frustration/anger, we have an over-abundance of stress and *"overload syndrome."*

Swanson's premise and book are all about the *root cause* of illness. Instead of just giving a pill for an ill, he gave a prescription for *margin*. Margin is what is missing in "overload syndrome."

Do you recognize any of these examples in your life?

- Activity overload
- Change overload
- Choice overload
- Commitment overload
- Debt overload
- Decision overload
- Expectation overload
- Fatigue overload
- Hurry overload
- Information overload

- Media overload
- Noise overload
- People overload
- Possession overload
- Technology overload
- Work overload

The formula for "margin" is straightforward: Power − Load = Margin

*Power* is made up of factors such as energy, skills, time, training, emotional and physical strength, faith, finances, and social support.

*Load* is made up of such factors as work, problems, obligations, commitments, expectations (internal and external), debt, deadlines, and interpersonal conflicts.

"When our load is *greater* than our power, we enter into negative *margin* status. That is, we are overloaded," writes Dr. Swenson. When our power is *greater* than our load, however, we have *margin*." Think of the margins in a book. If there were no margins—that is, no white space between paragraphs—and every page was filled with words from top to bottom, it would be overwhelming! (And nearly impossible to read.) Well, we live our lives like this. And the overload of stressors listed above have psychological symptoms, physical symptoms, behavioral symptoms, and yes, *burnout!*

In our modern world we are taught that we can do it all. Although I honestly believe that I "can do all things in Christ,"[7] I have also been taught by the scriptures that we "are not to walk faster than we can run,"[8] and that "our bodies are temples."[9] Running at the hastened pace we are living in today's world also has compound *negative* interest. This is what Dr. Swenson was seeing in patients, year after year! I've seen it, too.

I ran on fumes for years with little margin to even sleep. For those of us with rough, painful childhoods, the way many of us received any form of love or attention was by producing results of doing more and of being the best. If our culture does not set us up for this *"overload syndrome,"* then our own behavior of constantly proving our worth or disproving the negative stories in our head certainly will!

It's been a hard pattern to shift over the years. I've learned the hard way that, if we don't pay attention to the flashing dashboard lights represented by our symptoms (such as, this hurts, I'm exhausted, my brain is fogged), sooner or later our engines will burn out. God will get our attention, even if it means we are stopped by chronic fatigue or other health challenges.

Dr. Swenson shares that one of the reasons for this *"overload syndrome"* is that we all have a different tolerance level for busyness. We all have a different threshold before breakdown begins. Years ago, when I was pushing myself way past healthy margins, I did not know that I was one of the 20 percent of the population that are Highly Sensitive Persons (HSP). In essence, our nervous systems are also way more sensitive to stimuli of any kind, thus we can reach overload *sooner* than others. I have learned that what I need on a regular basis is more *margin*.

Margin is indeed the antidote to the *"overload syndrome."* I highly recommend this book if you notice that you have indications of overload syndrome in your life. Dr. Swenson gives several "prescriptions" to help us gain margin in our *emotional energy, physical energy, time, and finances*. For instance, if you want "time margin," his prescriptions are:

1. Expect the Unexpected
2. Learn to Say No
3. Turn off the Television
4. Prune the Activity Branches
5. Practice Simplicity and Contentment

6. Separate Time from Technology—This is why I practice a "digital sunset" and "digital sunrise" by keeping electronics off for at least an hour before bed and after I get up.
7. Short-Term Flurry Versus Long-Term Vision—I love the Power of 10 rule that we discussed in Chapter 7 to support me here.
8. Thank God
9. Sabotage Your Fuse Box (in other words, disconnect and get quiet)
10. Get Less Done but Do the Right Things
11. Enjoy Anticipation, Relish the Memories
12. Don't Rush Wisdom
13. For Type "A's" Only: stand in line
14. Create Buffer Zones
15. Plan for Free Time
16. Be Available

Note: if you are interested in learning more about Highly Sensitive Persons, see the Resources section.

# Meditate

Before I began a practice of daily meditation, I'll admit that I had misconceptions about its return on investment. My body, mind, and spirit needed the meditation, but I just didn't think that I could master it the way that the experts did. I assumed it would take years of practice for me to gain any benefit. Then, I took Brooke Snow's 40-day Christian Meditation Challenge. It was *life changing!* Really! The more I practice meditation, the more I love it. The more I learn about Epigenetics, the more I'm thrilled that I practice daily meditation. In fact, Herbert Benson, associate professor of medicine at Harvard Medical School, discovered that harmful genes leading to inflammation and free radical activity could be neutralized by a regular relaxation practice. That is awesome.[10]

Additionally, researchers[11] from Yale University School of Medicine found that meditating three times a week for six weeks improved endothelial (the lining of our vessels from head to toe) function and reduced blood pressure, resting heart rate, and the risk of heart disease.

Meditation has been shown to:
- Reduce stress
- Control anxiety
- Promote emotional health
- Enhance self-awareness
- Lengthen attention span
- Reduce age-related memory loss
- Generate kindness
- Help fight addictions
- Improve sleep
- Help control pain
- Decrease blood pressure
- Be accessible anywhere
- Be available for FREE

Why is this not being taught in medical schools? For that matter, why is meditation not being taught in elementary schools?

## Self-Mastery

What I have learned about meditation is that the point is *not* to be good at meditation, but to be master of myself—to act and not be acted upon;[12] to be the creator in my life, not a reactor! While the science of meditation is immense, with over 10,000 clinical studies on PubMed.gov alone, this is not the place to go into too much detail. But I do want to share a powerful explanation of the link between meditation and Creation Principles as taught to me by my expert mentor, Brooke Snow.

Meditation stands as a powerful tool for co-creation, especially when approached through a Christ-centered lens. It transcends mere personal devotion, evolving into a collaborative act with the Divine.

In the realm of spiritual creation through meditation, each aspect is encompassed: Visualization (SEE), Affirmation (SAY), Emotional connection (FEEL), Action (DO), and Transformation (BECOME). This process empowers you to rehearse desired manifestations through repetition, effectively rewiring the subconscious. By adhering to these principles, meditation becomes a profound means of shifting from negativity to positivity, nurturing one's core identity.

Fundamentally, meditation is about creation, aiming to align our lives with the divine blueprint of our being. This requires a tangible shift in mindset. Whether it's cultivating patience, tranquility, or fostering deeper love and connection, meditation offers a platform to mentally and physically rehearse these desired states. Through envisioning, affirming, feeling, and acting upon them, internal transformation occurs, reinforcing the mind-body connection.

With persistent practice, these patterns integrate deeply into one's being, thereby enhancing embodiment. The true benefit arises when responses become instinctual; virtues like patience and connection become innate qualities rather than conscious efforts. Through consistent rehearsal, a new mindset is not only created but fully embodied.

Meditation serves as a potent tool for co-creation. When adopting a Christ-centered approach to meditation, it becomes not only a practice of personal devotion but also an act of collaborative creation with the Divine.

Now, doesn't that inspire to you try meditation, even a few minutes each morning to create your day? I have found meditation to be so incredibly supportive in creating new habits and changing old self-sabotaging patterns. As I've highlighted throughout this book, emotions can get buried deep in our bodies, including our DNA. Wouldn't it be a better practice to clear those emotions through meditation? I have been thrilled with the "dress rehearsal" effect of creating my day, even my interactions, through meditation in the morning. I have been calmed and feel closer to Christ as I rehearse the day—including my potential interactions and through "review-type" meditation in the evening. I can even rehearse a "do-over." This has made my daily repentance process a joy. Who needs to be carrying the baggage of guilt or upset? No one!

See my Resources section for meditation apps that I recommend.

# Let Go

As I've shared earlier, I struggled with fatigue for many years. Yes, I had some real physiological stressors that were sucking the energy right out of me, yet it was *more* than a physiological issue. It wasn't until I started doing 12-step recovery work for codependency that I felt totally revitalized. I had no idea how people pleasing, controlling, and perfectionism were sucking the life out of me! As one of my fellow recovery sista's said, "I *didn't know, until I knew.*"

I did not grow up with addiction, per say. I didn't have any substance abuse or other abuse issues that one might commonly see (food, work, sex, shopping), but addiction to drama, dysfunction, abuse, and toxic shaming were certainly present. In Jeanette Elizabeth Menter's illuminating book, *You're Not Crazy, You're Codependent*,[13] she teaches that the four most common causes of codependency in personal development are:

- Addiction
- Abuse
- Toxic shame-based treatment
- Trauma

Do any of these resonate with you? If not, here are some other characteristics of people with codependency that might sound or feel familiar:

- An exaggerated sense of responsibility for the actions of others
- A tendency to confuse love and pity, with the tendency to "love" people who we can pity and rescue
- A tendency to do more than our share, all the time
- A tendency to become hurt when people don't recognize our efforts
- An unhealthy dependence on relationships. The codependent will do anything to hold on to a relationship; to avoid the feeling of abandonment
- An extreme need for approval and recognition
- A sense of guilt when asserting ourselves
- A compelling need to control others
- Lack of trust in self and/or others
- Fear of being abandoned or alone
- Difficulty identifying feelings
- Rigidity/difficulty adjusting to change
- Problems with intimacy/boundaries
- Chronic anger
- Lying/dishonesty
- Poor communications
- Difficulty making decisions

I must admit that I could check off quite a few of these before I began my recovery journey. False notions that you can control the outcome by people pleasing and being perfect are exhausting!

Lack of boundaries and doing too much for other people are also exhausting! Chronic anger and resentment suck the life out of you and keep you resonating at a very low level, which is also exhausting!

Ann Landers once said:

> "Some people believe holding on and hanging in there are signs of great strength. However, there are times when it takes much more strength to know when to let go and then do it."

Digging in and doing the hard healing work of recovery has been worth the effort. The *freedom* of "Letting Go" has been divine. Yes, it takes practice and daily effort, yet the renewed vitality and joy have been worth it!

By beginning to understand how powerless I am over the actions and lives of others and trusting God on a whole new level, my spiritual, emotional, mental, and physical health has been transformed! Really understanding the "Serenity Prayer" in my bones has allowed me to heal on every level.

> "God grant me the **Serenity** to accept the things I cannot change, the **Courage** to change the things I can, and the **Wisdom** to know the difference. Living one day at a time, trusting that You (God) will make all things right if I surrender to Your (His) will." *Parentheses added*

Let's take a deep dive into these amazing words and see the energetic frequency of each of these words.

**Serenity** – Serenity means the state of being calm, peaceful and untroubled. Antonyms for serenity are agitation, turbulence, turmoil, unrest, and upheaval. Would you prefer to resonate at the frequency of calm and peace or turmoil and unrest?

**Accept** – Acceptance means to receive or take responsibility. Antonyms are to reject, deny, disallow and forfeit. I fought acceptance for years by fighting reality. Do you know the old saying "kicking against the bricks"? It hurts! Byron Katie so powerfully states, "When you argue against reality, you lose, but only 100% of the time." That's a lot of wasted energy. When we resist, it just persists. Acceptance is a much gentler energy for our bodies to manage.

**Courage** – Courage is the ability to do something that frightens us and using strength in the face of pain or grief. It's a choice and willingness to deal with agony, pain, danger, uncertainty, and intimidation. Harold B. Lee, one of my heroes years ago, suggested that we study the "Serenity Prayer" and that "courage is an affair of the Spirit." The antithesis of courage is fear, cowardice, and faintheartedness. Would you rather resonate with courage or fear?

**Wisdom** – Wisdom means the knowledge of what is true or right coupled with just judgment as to action, sagacity, discernment, or insight. The antithesis of wisdom is ignorance, stupidity, thoughtlessness, and imprudence. Where would you rather resonate?

Notice your own body whenever you articulate these or other negative words. See what happens to your physiology. Expressed verbally, the antonyms of serenity, accept, courage, and wisdom attract more of the same and, as such, an encounter with "Murphy's Law."

By contrast, higher-frequency emotions and words—like Serenity, Acceptance, Courage, and Wisdom—can create a noticeable and immediate shift in your energy. Try it for yourself: speak or read the Serenity Prayer and notice the difference in how you feel. As you begin to incorporate more high-frequency words in your conversations, you will vibrate at a higher emotional frequency, and your experiences will match those levels.

As I have daily practiced the art of recovery, I have learned to exchange codependency for *divine* dependency. As I completely rely upon my Father in Heaven (and for you it may be whatever Higher Power you choose), then I have a greater capacity to access and maintain emotional and spiritual health.

## Be Grateful

When my body was so sick, being grateful for an amazing team of functional health providers as well as the incredible curriculum that God was teaching me, I was able to snap out of the "woe is me" attitude and step into what I needed to do to continue my healing journey. Gratitude is an amazing tool to quickly accomplish a mental shift for whatever may be troubling you.

In fact, gratitude is a transformative emotion that influences our emotional and mental well-being, our spiritual connectivity, and our physical health. Its epigenetic impact supplies us with a scientific foundation for embracing gratitude as a potent instrument for inner tranquility and heightened vitality. "Our thoughts change our biochemistry, which changes the behavior of our cells," stated Bruce Lipton, PhD.[14] Wow—that's a lot of epigenetic power! By fostering gratitude in our lives, we not only experience enhanced emotional well-being, but we also unlock pathways to a more profound sense of purpose and fulfillment in our spiritual journey.

> "Gratitude unlocks the fullness of life. It turns what we
> have into enough, and more. It turns denial into acceptance,
> chaos into order, confusion into clarity. It can turn a meal
> into a feast, a house into a home, a stranger into a friend."
> ~Melody Beattie

## The science of gratitude

A small, randomized, controlled clinical trial[15] of 35- to 50-year-old women was done to evaluate the impact of gratitude on both neural activity and inflammatory markers. The women who were in the intervention and gratitude-practicing arm of the study were found to have larger reductions in amygdala reactivity in the brain. The amygdala is what gets fired when we are under stress or in a sympathetic, fight or flight experience. Because these women practiced the gratitude tasks, this area of the brain was calmer than those of the control subjects. Think of that the next time you're stressed. Those women who had a calmer, less reactive amygdala also had lower inflammatory markers (TNF-α & IL-6). By practicing meditation and combining it with the power of gratitude, imagine the benefits to your spiritual, mental, emotional, and physical bodies! Other studies reveal that instituting the practice of daily gratitude not only creates improvements in sleep, but also causes significant reductions in diastolic blood pressure.[16]

At the Institute of HeartMath,[17] a group of prestigious and internationally recognized leaders in physics, biophysics, astrophysics, education, mathematics, engineering, cardiology, biofeedback, and psychology (among other disciplines) have been doing brilliant work on heart coherence and its impact on the brain. According to Rollin McCraty, PhD, director of research at HeartMath, their research has demonstrated that when an individual experiences profoundly positive emotions such as gratitude, love, or appreciation, the heart transmits a distinct message, influencing the nature of signals dispatched to the brain. The HeartMath team also discovered that individuals experiencing gratitude exhibited a notable decrease in cortisol, the stress hormone. These participants demonstrated enhanced cardiac function and displayed greater resilience in the face of emotional setbacks and negative experiences.

Other cardiovascular factors impacted by gratitude include improved High Density Lipoproteins (HDL) or healthy cholesterol, decreased Low Density Lipoproteins (LDL) or bad cholesterol, and reduced blood pressure. That's just from having an attitude of gratitude!

Additional studies done to examine the physical effects of gratitude include a pilot study published in the journal *Psychosomatic Medicine*.[18] This study with Stage B heart failure patients divided participants into two groups to examine whether gratitude journaling improved biomarkers related to heart failure prognosis. After eight weeks, those that were writing in a gratitude journal showed *both* a reduced inflammatory biomarker index score over time as well as significant improvements in heart rate variability (HRV). HRV is an indicator of our balance between the Sympathetic Nervous System (SNS) and our Parasympathetic Nervous System (PSNS). When our PSNS activity rises, then our HRV score will, too. The higher the better, unless you do indeed have a saber tooth tiger running after you.

Gratitude has been shown to improve sleep, decrease pain, and improve immune function, too. We cannot dwell in gratitude and worry at the same time; therefore, when we are practicing gratitude our stress hormone cortisol can decrease. This in turn has a profound impact on our hormone balance. As you recall from Chapter 14, a reduction in cortisol levels can help diminish the risk of estrogen dominance, which is known to have far-reaching effects on us physically, mentally, and emotionally.

Dr. Joe Dispenza—Lipton's colleague in this amazing work of Epigenetics and the power of our thoughts—had done extensive research looking at the effect of using higher-level emotions to heal our bodies. Dispenza states, ". . . when we feel an elevated emotion (like gratitude), we can begin to signal our genes ahead of the environment." He also states that "Gratitude is the ultimate source of receiving."[19]

Now that I've shared how gratitude can impact your physical health, let's look at many other amazing benefits of gratitude.

## The emotional impact of gratitude

"Gratitude is the healthiest of all human emotions," proclaimed Zig Ziglar. Without a doubt, gratitude transcends momentary feelings and leaves a lasting impact on our emotional well-being. Regular expressions of gratitude possess the potential to influence the expression of stress-related genes, which in turn makes us more resilient to conditions like anxiety and depression. Engaging in gratitude practices not only regulates stress hormones, thereby alleviating fear and anxiety, but also boosts levels of serotonin and dopamine, the neurotransmitters linked to happiness. Furthermore, it contributes to the formation of new neural pathways, cultivating an elevated sense of happiness.

The incorporation of gratitude practices into our lives has been correlated with heightened levels of empathy and pro-social behavior. A study from 2017[20,21] uncovered that individuals who routinely engaged in gratitude exercises were more inclined to display pro-social behaviors, including acts of kindness and compassion. This emotional dimension of gratitude enriches our connections with others and nurtures more meaningful relationships. Additionally, a study involving undergraduate students found that practicing gratitude served to diminish feelings of envy.[22]

## The spiritual impact of gratitude

Gratitude isn't just about feeling good; it's about deepening our spiritual connection and finding more meaning in life.

Gratitude stands as a fundamental pillar in numerous spiritual and religious traditions. By directing our attention to appreciating "every good gift and every perfect gift from above"[23] we are prompted to recognize that these gifts emanate from the Heavenly Father, who possesses individual awareness of each of us. The practice of gratitude serves as a poignant reminder that divine benevolence seeks to bestow abundance across all facets of our lives.

Furthermore, gratitude rituals have been associated with heightened sensations of interconnectedness and transcendence. A study[24] featured in the *Handbook of Positive Psychology, Religion and Spirituality* unveiled that those individuals who consistently participated in gratitude exercises reported elevated levels of spirituality and a profound sense of connection to something greater than themselves.

What if we were to feel gratitude for the people we loved? What if we recited some of their beautiful traits before we conversed with them? Do you think it would change your interactions? I think it would change marriages, families, communities, and the world! According to the HeartMath team, this could lead to not only coherence in our families, but even global coherence.

# Cultivating Gratitude

The three practices I describe below have transformed my level of gratitude, and therefore my life. All three are simple to do, and I hope you consider adopting at least one of them to uplevel your ability to cultivate gratitude.

## What's awesome about this?

The next time you're faced with a difficult or disappointing situation or idea, ask yourself: "*What's Awesome About This?*" I acquired this insightful practice during my 2021 Creation Coach certification program. Whenever faced with less-than-ideal situations, I've adopted the habit of asking myself, "What's awesome about this?" Over time, this mental exercise has strengthened, much like a muscle. While in the past it might have taken several minutes or even an hour to pose this question to myself, now I can swiftly shift my mindset within seconds.

For example, one day I had just completed a blog post, and it was ready to send to my virtual assistant. Unexpectedly, I lost the entire content. Deleted, gone, beyond retrieval. This hadn't happened in years, and my initial reaction was a distressing, "Oh NO! Now what?!" However, within two minutes, I redirected my thinking to, *What's awesome about this?* This rapid shift not only helped calm my stress hormones, but it also prompted me to contemplate potential hidden benefits. What turned out to be the silver lining in this situation? To my surprise and delight, starting over from scratch sparked new inspiration.

## Gratitude journaling

For years, the idea of maintaining a gratitude journal lingered in my thoughts. I was aware that this practice not only alleviates stress but also enhances sleep quality and cultivates emotional awareness.[25] I was stuck trying to find a habit that would stick. The key for me was finding a more straightforward way to journal. Once I discovered the Day One App, a fantastic application that synchronizes seamlessly across all my devices, I was able to establish consistency. Setting a goal to jot down—or in my case, sometime dictate—three bullet points each day just before bedtime, I harnessed the power of neuroplasticity, aiming to forge a new neural pathway dedicated to gratitude. Over time, those initial three bullet points evolved into seven. Eventually, I found myself dictating entire paragraphs, sometimes even in the early morning.

The true payoff of this newfound habit became evident during my divorce. By consciously counting my blessings throughout the day and taking a few moments to dictate them, I managed to maintain a higher frequency of gratitude amidst the most intense challenge of my life. While I experienced profound grief throughout this journey, the daily focus on gratitude empowered me with a much more optimistic perspective on my future, surpassing the grip of anger and resentment. I was able to SEE beyond the immediate grief and trauma and create a very different experience of serenity.

## Mindfulness and meditation

Once again, I found myself contemplating a habit that I had envisioned starting "someday." The ideal moment finally presented itself during the pandemic quarantine. As I initiated a daily meditation routine, my thoughts gradually slowed, and a heightened sense of awareness emerged. Mindfulness practices proved instrumental in connecting with the present moment and recognizing the blessings woven into my life. Starting my day with meditation and expressions of gratitude toward God, as we co-create the day together, automatically places me in a state of gratitude. In turn, this primed me to observe and appreciate joy and abundance throughout the day, providing rich material for reflection in my evening journaling.

Can you see how these three simple habits work together to increase gratitude and resilience?

Gratitude works to reshape our hearts and souls, thereby fostering greater compassion, interconnectedness, and spiritual enrichment. Not only that, but gratitude also holds the potential to mitigate inflammation, enhance cognitive function, and amplify overall feelings of vitality. According to Dr. Lipton and Dr. Dispenza, these transformations extend to our gene expression and physical health. Therefore, become part of the gratitude movement and embark on the journey to transform your body, mind, and spirit. You'll be grateful you did!

## Consider This

- Where are you experiencing "overload syndrome" in your life?

- What's a simple floor you could create to help you begin to create some "margin" in your life?

- What's a simple meditation practice you could try for five minutes, either every morning, at lunch, or before bed?

- What practice can you add to your life to cultivate more gratitude?

# Seventeen

# Be Your Best Self

> "Happiness is the new rich. Inner peace is the new success.
> Health is the new wealth. Kindness is the new cool."
>
> ~ANONYMOUS

As we continue to learn to employ the Creation Principles to embody true vitality, it is important for us to examine the "SAY" and "FEEL" aspects of the process. As we embrace the attributes of being present, forgiving, and making amends, we have greater capacity to be joyful! Being our human capacities will create the space to manifest our divine nature in a greater way and live our entire spiritual, emotional, mental, and physical selves wholeheartedly.

## Be Present

In the relentless rhythm of modern life, where the incessant demands of work, relationships, and personal responsibilities can feel overwhelming, the concept of vitality stands out as a beacon of hope—a reminder that amidst the chaos, we possess an innate wellspring of energy waiting to be tapped. The modern dilemma of perpetual multitasking and digital distraction often leaves

> *"The Present is the point at which Time touches eternity."*
>
> ~C.S. LEWIS

us physically present but mentally absent, robbing us of the richness inherent in each passing moment. In the pursuit of a vibrant and fulfilling life, one of the most transformative keys lies in the power of being present.

## The modern dilemma: A life on autopilot

How often do you find yourself going from one room to the next and forgetting what you went there for? If you're aging (and all of us are), there may be hormonal imbalance or cognitive decline that may be a contributing factor, but often we have just slipped into autopilot mode, where routine tasks unfold mechanically, and the nuances of our experiences are lost in the shuffle.

Our vitality is intricately tied to our ability to break free from the chains of mindless routine and engage *fully* with the present. The present moment, often underestimated in its significance, becomes the canvas upon which the masterpiece of our lives is painted. The present is where we can experience true joy.

## The essence of presence: A gateway to vitality

When we talk about the power of being present, we refer to a conscious and intentional focus on the current moment. It is an art that requires practice—an art that, when mastered, can transform the mundane into the extraordinary.

At the heart of being present is mindfulness—a state of heightened awareness and attention to the present experience. I'm the first to admit that, for many years, I lived on autopilot running around like a chicken with my head cut off. I was doing, doing, doing. I had been rewarded for productivity, and I was good at it. However, I was often not present.

Jon Kabot- Zinn practiced at the University of Massachusetts Medical Center where I did my first graduate work. I have an autographed copy of his book *Full Catastrophe Living*,[1] yet I didn't open his book until years later. I was too busy *doing* rather than *being* to even consider mindfulness or meditation. What I eventually learned is that mindfulness is not about erasing the past or ignoring the future; rather, it is about acknowledging them without being consumed by them. It is a deliberate choice to inhabit the now, recognizing that life's most profound moments unfold in the present.

When we choose to be fully present, we open ourselves up to the richness of each moment. It's a conscious decision to be attentive to the sights, sounds, and sensations that surround us. The sunlight filtering through the leaves, the laughter of children playing, the subtle fragrance of blooming flowers—these are not just details; they are the building blocks of a vibrant and interconnected tapestry.

> "Mindfulness is like a stethoscope you hold to your heart; it lets you know how you're feeling in a particular moment, so you can figure out what to do next."
>
> ~ANONYMOUS

In our quest for vitality, this heightened awareness becomes a source of renewed energy. This connection with the present moment acts as a wellspring, infusing us with a sense of aliveness that transcends the physical realm.

Moreover, the richness of each moment serves as a counterbalance to the monotony and stressors of daily life. The practice of being present allows us to step off the perpetual treadmill of worries about the past or anxieties about the future. In doing so, we create a space for tranquility to emerge—a tranquil space where our minds can rest and rejuvenate.

## Mindful living and stress reduction

When we are fully present, stress loses its grip. The mind, unburdened by the weight of past regrets or future uncertainties, finds respite in the now. This mental liberation has cascading effects on the body, influencing everything from heart rate to immune function, as we discussed in Chapter 16. Research has shown that mindfulness practices, which emphasize being present, can lead to measurable reductions in stress hormones and improvements in overall health.

For instance, a study conducted by Kabat-Zinn and colleagues in 2003[2] demonstrated that participants in a mindfulness-based, stress-reduction program exhibited significant reductions in stress and improvements in psychological well-being. Furthermore, research[3] indicates that mindfulness meditation can positively impact the autonomic nervous system, contributing to stress reduction and improved overall health. Personally, I love how my meditation practice prepares me for my daily interactions with others. I can have a dress rehearsal for how I want to show up, and how I want to be present with others.

## Deepening connections in relationships

Presence in relationships is not merely about proximity; it is about a quality of attention that transcends the superficial. When we are fully present with someone, we communicate on a deeper level—a level where understanding, empathy, and connection thrive. In the rush of modern life, the simple act of truly listening to a friend, partner, or family member becomes a rare and precious gift.

The physiological benefits of deep connections extend beyond emotional well-being. Research in the field of psychoneuroimmunology suggests that positive social interactions, facilitated by being present and engaged in relationships, can enhance immune function and contribute to overall health.[4]

Moreover, the impact of presence extends beyond our immediate relationships; it ripples outward, influencing the collective consciousness of communities and societies. By embodying the values of presence—compassion, understanding, and mutual respect—we contribute to the creation of a more connected and vibrant world.

## The present as a portal for personal growth

In the unfolding tapestry of our lives, each moment presents an opportunity for learning, resilience, and transformation. When we confront challenges with a spirit of presence, we engage with them authentically. Instead of viewing difficulties as obstacles to be avoided, we see them as invitations for growth. The present moment becomes a classroom where we learn about ourselves— our strengths, our limitations, and our capacity for resilience.

Celebrating victories, both big and small, is equally essential on this journey of self-discovery. By acknowledging and savoring our achievements in the present, we cultivate a positive and empowering narrative that propels us forward. The power of being present in moments of triumph allows us to fully absorb the joy and satisfaction that accompanies success.

## Cultivating the habit of presence

Embracing the power of being present is not a one-time endeavor; it is a lifelong practice that requires cultivation and commitment. Fortunately, there are various mindfulness techniques and practices that serve as gateways to presence.

- **Mindful Breathing:** One of the simplest yet most powerful techniques is mindful breathing. By directing our attention to the rhythmic inhaling and exhaling of breath, we anchor ourselves in the present moment. The breath becomes a reliable anchor, grounding us in the now.
- **Body Scan Meditation:** This practice involves systematically directing attention to different parts of the body, cultivating awareness of sensations and promoting a deep sense of relaxation. The body scan is an effective tool for bringing the mind into the present moment.

- **Mindful Walking:** Engaging in mindful walking is another way to integrate presence into everyday life. Whether in nature or amidst the urban landscape, walking mindfully involves paying attention to each step, the sensation of movement, and the surrounding environment.
- **Gratitude Practice:** Here we are again, back to gratitude. Gratitude is also a potent catalyst for presence. Taking a few moments each day to reflect on and express gratitude for the positive aspects of our lives shifts our focus from what is lacking to what is abundant, fostering a sense of contentment in the present.

Embark on your journey to vitality with an open heart and an attentive mind. You will find that it is in the *present* where the magic of vitality unfolds, inviting you to live a life that is not just lived, but truly experienced.

## Be Forgiving

When I attended the August 2019 presentation by Bruce Lipton, PhD, the entire audience was riveted on his every word for 90 minutes. When his presentation was complete, the standing ovations over, and the mics off, he then surprised us all as he hopped back up on the stage and said, "I have one more thing to say." The room fell silent enough to hear a pin drop. I will never forget the words that came from his mouth: "Cancer is caused by the lack of forgiveness." Wow! Lipton, a brilliant medical school professor of cellular biology, whose entire career was changed as he began to understand quantum physics, was reinforcing how our emotions, especially our toxic unhealed emotions, can cause the most dreaded of dis-eases.

Let me clarify my point in sharing Lipton's quote. I am *not* saying that all cancers are caused by the lack of forgiveness, nor is Dr. Lipton. I'm certain that my dear friend's precious little Madi, who died at the age 4, did not have forgiveness issues that caused her cancer. You may also know of young children or even the most kind-hearted adults who do not have an ounce of anger or revenge in their bodies and yet still got cancer. However, Lipton's point is that we may all want to consider the vibration of our thoughts and feelings and the impact on our health.

## The vibration of negative emotions

In Chapter 16, I discussed the importance of letting go as well as the science from Candace Pert, PhD. Remember, our emotions most definitely impact our bodies and can become buried on a cellular level, even down to the DNA.

### THE MHz OF EMOTIONS

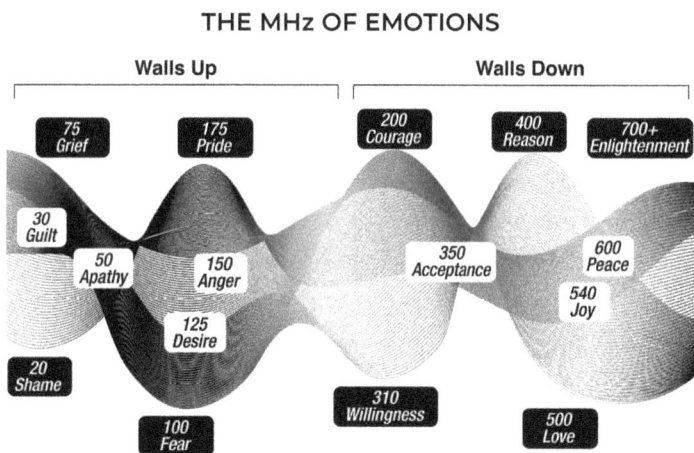

Figure 3: Note the frequency (MHz) of
positive and negative emotions

Emotions such as love, joy, peace, and enlightenment resonate at a very high level (500 MHz – 700+ MHz) and are wonderful for your state of health and vitality. Pride, anger, fear, grief, apathy, guilt, and shame progressively drop in MHz down from 175 MHz to 20Mhz. Disease starts at approximately 58 MHz, and cancer starts at 42 MHz. When we are living with feelings of anger, bitterness, revenge, and resentment, we are bound to experience the profound negative effects on our body.

In much of today's popular culture, the virtues of forgiveness and kindness are belittled, while ridicule, anger, and harsh criticism are encouraged. If we are not careful, we can fall prey to these habits within our own homes and families and soon find ourselves criticizing our spouse, our children, and our extended family members.

## Religion and science agree:
## We have been commanded to forgive

Forgiveness is an age-old practice central to the teachings of many of the world's religions. In Islam, forgiveness suggests alignment with Allah. In Judaism, acts of Atonement (Teshuva) are expected for wrongdoing. And in Christianity, Christ is the supreme example of forgiveness.

The great crowning love of the Jesus Christ was expressed when, in His dying agony, He cried out, "Father, forgive them; for they know not what they do."[5] Christ taught, "But I say unto you, love your enemies, bless them that curse you, do good to them that hate you, and pray for them which despitefully use you, and persecute you."[6] There are even stronger commands in scripture: "...but of you it is required to forgive all men"[7] and if we do not forgive, *we* will be the one that "hath brought *himself (ourselves)* under condemnation."[8] (Italics added)

Even if it appears that another may be deserving of our resentment or hatred, none of us can afford to pay the price of resenting or hating because of what it does to ourselves. If we have felt the gnawing, caustic nature of these emotions, we need to realize they can harm us if left unchecked.

## What Is forgiveness?

Forgiveness is freeing up and putting to better use the energy once consumed by holding grudges, harboring resentments, and nursing unhealed wounds. It is rediscovering the strengths we always had and reallocating our limitless capacity to understand and accept other people and ourselves. As one of my mentors, Alison Armstrong, said years go: "Forgiveness is giving as before."

Forgiveness does not deny that we have been hurt. On the contrary, we have to admit that we have been hurt and that we have a right to feel hurt, angry, or resentful. Unwillingness to admit that we have been hurt is one of the major impediments to forgiving.

Forgiveness does not require us to accept or tolerate evil. It does not require us to ignore the wrong that we see in the world around us or in our own lives. But as we fight against sin, we must not allow hatred or anger to control our thoughts or actions.

Joanna North of Great Britain gave this apt definition of forgiveness: "When unjustly hurt by another, we forgive when we overcome the resentment toward the offender, not by denying our right to the resentment, but instead by trying to offer the wrongdoer compassion, benevolence, and love; as we give these, we as forgivers, realize that the offender does not necessarily have a right to such gifts."[9]

## What is anger?

Anger is the primary and, in many ways, *proper* response to injury. Resentment, on the hand, involves re-feeling the original anger. We remember the injury and "re-feel the emotions surrounding our heart. Anger is like a flame; resentment is like a hot coal." Anger can be healthy to release, yet too much anger frequently expressed can suck the vitality right out of you—or even be deadly.[10,11]

As early as 1939, there are clinical studies revealing that anger has an impact on our physiology. Franz Alexander, MD, showed that *young college students* who had borderline high blood pressure showed higher levels of passive anger than those with normal blood pressure.

In my years working as a Nurse Practitioner in Cardiology, I remember the big news about the best-selling *Anger Kills*[12] by Virginia and Redford Williams. This book focused on the "Type A personality" and the hypothesized link to heart disease. As scientists dug deeper, the evidence clearly revealed that it was hostility, cynicism, mistrust, intense angry feelings, and patterns of aggressive behavior that create the *real* health risk.

As decades of research have followed, there is more evidence revealing the devastation that chronic anger and hostility have on our health and vitality.

"Anger is a form of stress, and so when we hold on to anger it is as though we are turning on the body's stress response, or fight or flight response, chronically. We know that turning on this response chronically leads to wear and tear on the body," said Neda Gould, a clinical psychologist and assistant professor of psychiatry and behavioral sciences at Johns Hopkins University School of Medicine. She continues, "It may not be surprising that when we engage in the act of forgiveness, we can begin to turn off the stress response and the physiological changes that accompany it."[13]

Karen Swartz, M.D., director of Mood Disorders Adult Consultation Clinic at The Johns Hopkins Hospital puts it this way, "There is an enormous physical burden to being hurt and disappointed. Chronic anger puts you into a fight-or-flight mode, which results in numerous changes in heart rate, blood pressure and immune response.[14] Those changes, then, increase the risk of depression, heart disease and diabetes, among other conditions. Forgiveness, however, calms stress levels, leading to improved health."

Additionally, forgiveness is shown to improve cholesterol levels and sleep, while reducing pain, blood pressure, and levels of anxiety, depression, and stress. The bonus—research points to an increase in the forgiveness-health connection as you age.[15]

## The power of forgiveness

There are two sides to forgiveness: decisional and emotional. Decisional forgiveness involves a conscious choice to replace ill will with good will. "You no longer wish bad things to happen to that individual," says Dr. Tyler VanderWeele, co-director of the Initiative on Health, Religion, and Spirituality at the Harvard T.H. Chan School of Public Health. "This is often quicker and easier to accomplish."[16]

For emotional forgiveness, you move away from those negative feelings and no longer dwell on the wrongdoing. "Emotional forgiveness is much harder and takes longer, as it's common for those feelings to return on a regular basis," says Dr. VanderWeele. "This often happens when you think about the offender, or something triggers the memory, or you still suffer from the adverse consequences of the action."[17]

As we've discussed, practicing forgiveness can have powerful health benefits. Observational studies, and even some randomized trials, suggest that forgiveness is associated with lower levels of depression, anxiety, and hostility; reduced substance abuse; higher self-esteem; and greater life satisfaction. Yet, forgiving people is *not* always easy.

## Forgiveness is a choice

Robert Enrich, PhD, reiterates in his book that *Forgiveness is a Choice*.[18] Forgiving begins with pain, and we have a right to our feelings. We acknowledge that the offense was unfair; we have a moral right to anger; and forgiveness requires giving up something to which we have a right—namely our anger or resentment.

Forgiving is an act of mercy toward the offender. The ability to forgive—to transform anger and resentment into hope and healing, said James E. Faust[19]—"can indeed be a restorative and healing act requiring faith." The following story showcases how restorative and healing it *can* be.

A 32-year-old milk truck driver lived with his family in their Nickel Mines community. He was not Amish, but his pickup route took him to many Amish dairy farms, where he became known as the quiet milkman. On October 2, 2006, he suddenly lost all reason and control. In his tormented mind, he blamed God for the death of his first child and some unsubstantiated memories. He stormed into the Amish school without any provocation, released the boys and adults, and tied up the 10 girls. He shot the girls, killing five and wounding five. Then he took his own life.[20]

This shocking violence caused great anguish among the Amish but no anger. There was hurt but no hate. Their forgiveness was immediate. Collectively they began to reach out to the milkman's suffering family. As the milkman's family gathered in his home the day after the shootings, an Amish neighbor came over, wrapped his arms around the father of the dead gunman, and said, "We will forgive you." Amish leaders visited the milkman's wife and children to extend their sympathy, their forgiveness, their help, and their love. About half of the mourners at the milkman's funeral were Amish. In turn, the Amish invited the milkman's family to attend the funeral services of the girls

*"We can find all manner of reasons for postponing forgiveness. One of these reasons is waiting for the wrongdoers to repent before we forgive them. Yet such a delay causes us to forfeit the peace and happiness that could be ours. The folly of rehashing long-past hurts does not bring happiness."*

~JAMES E. FAUST

who had been killed. A remarkable peace settled on the Amish as their faith sustained them during this crisis.

One local resident very eloquently summed up the aftermath of this tragedy when he said, "We were all speaking the same language, and not just English, but a language of caring, a language of community, [and] a language of service. And, yes, a language of forgiveness."

Clearly, there is plenty of scriptural and scientific evidence to show that forgiveness can indeed bless us spiritually, emotionally, mentally, and even physically, as hatred stunts our spiritual growth.

## How to forgive

Forgiveness does *not* mean that we deny an injury or harm has occurred. In fact, when Christ returned in His resurrected body, he left the wounds in His hands and feet as a reminder of the pain that He endured and overcame!

Archbishop and Nobel Prize winner Desmond Tutu, and his daughter Mpho, have written a glorious book on forgiveness entitled *The Book of Forgiving – The Fourfold Path for Healing Ourselves and Our World*.[21] They state that healing demands that we indeed identify behavior that is hurtful, shameful, abusive, and demeaning in any way. It must be brought info fierce light. The truth can be brutal, and it may actually exacerbate the hurt; however, "if we want real forgiveness, real healing, we must face the real injury."

They further clarify that:

- Forgiveness is not weakness. It is not spineless.
  It is not for the faint of heart.
- Forgiving does not mean being spineless;
  nor does it mean one doesn't get angry.
- Forgiveness is not a subversion to justice.
- Forgiveness is not forgetting.
- Forgiveness is not easy.

## The path of forgiveness

The Tutus state that revenge and forgiveness start at the same point, with hurt, harm, or loss, and are then followed by pain! The CHOICE then comes. The choice to *hurt* or the choice to *heal*.

In choosing the hurt, we have to reject the offender's shared humanity. We have to objectify them. Once they are rejected, the revenge, retaliation, and even violence is easy to justify. The Tutus explain in their book that the path to forgiveness entails telling the truth. Really telling the story, over and over again, to get it all out. The hurts do need to be named. It may mean telling the story to beloved friends and family, a supportive therapist, a 12-step recovery group, or even writing the details in a journal. In fact, most of the healing books I have read suggest journaling in detail.

After naming the hurt, now we go about the granting of forgiveness. Again, this may be decisional forgiveness to begin. Then we can pray to God for the help to release the emotional wounds and thus emotionally forgive. The reward: then, we can choose if we want to renew or release the relationship. Forgiveness does not mean we need to re-enter an abusive relationship. Yet the forgiveness will release *you* to move on to create the life that you are entitled to enjoy.

## Forgiveness is a lifelong practice

We are all going to experience hurt and pain in our lives. What will our response be when we are offended, misunderstood, or unfairly or unkindly treated? What will it be when we are sinned against, made an offender for a word, falsely accused, passed over, hurt by those we love, our offerings rejected? Do we resent, become bitter, hold a grudge? Or do we resolve the problem if we can, forgive, and rid ourselves of the burden?

The choice is indeed ours—whether we are going to be trapped into an endless loop of anger, resentment, bitterness, and victimhood, or we are going to choose to release, forgive, and not let the offender take another precious moment of our lives!

Forgiveness opens the door to peace *between* people and the space for peace *within* each person. The victim cannot have peace without forgiving. The perpetrator will not have genuine peace while unforgiven. The invitation to forgive is an invitation to search out the perpetrator's humanity. Reflect again on the Amish people. These people clearly *chose* forgiveness, and the effect was widespread. I would venture to say it was even immediate for all that were involved. What if we all followed their beautiful example?

Breaking negative cycles is paramount to raising your emotional state to mainly experiencing higher frequency vibration emotions such as joy, love, and acceptance. This begins by using our *will* to choose that we no longer wish to engage in such low vibrational energy.

Karol Truman's, DC, paramount book, *Feelings Buried Alive Never Die*,[22] clearly reinforces the work of Dr. Bruce Lipton and Dr. Candace Pert—that we need to detox the toxic, low-vibrational emotions if we want to live a life of vitality and fulfill the measure of our creation.

When I experienced the deepest hurt in my entire life, I'm grateful that the *first* thought that God blessed me with was, "This too shall be Redeemed, Lori." Our hurts, our pains, our sufferings, all of it can be consecrated for good if we ask God for His blessing.

We have all heard "Hurt people, *hurt* people." But what if we changed that and said, "healed people, *heal* people"? What if we all did the healing work necessary to vibrate at a higher level? As the Tutus proclaim, it would not just change our families and neighborhoods but the whole world!

# Make Amends that Work

Have you ever tried to apologize, or make amends, and it just didn't land? The person on the other end was *not* hearing the apology. Perhaps you felt that you'd tried until you were "blue in the face," and it still just didn't go anywhere. That could be because you were not speaking *their* apology language. This is where a new tool can help.

Gary Chapman, a well-known author, speaker, and counselor, is perhaps best known for his book *The Five Love Languages*. He has since written about apologies and forgiveness in relationships, outlining what he calls the "five apology languages." In his book *The 5 Apology Languages: The Secret to Healthy Relationships"* co-authored with Jennifer Thomas, Chapman presents a framework for understanding how individuals give and receive apologies.[23]

## The languages of apologies

Chapman's concept of apology languages can be applied to various types of relationships, including romantic partnerships, friendships, family dynamics, and professional interactions. By identifying and speaking the appropriate apology language, individuals can strengthen their connections, rebuild trust, and foster healthier relationships overall. Let's take a look at these five apology languages.

### 1. Expressing regret

Expressing regret is more than just saying "I'm sorry." It involves acknowledging the specific hurt or harm caused by one's actions and demonstrating genuine remorse for it. This apology language requires empathy and understanding of the other person's feelings. When someone values the expression of regret, they seek validation that the other party truly comprehends the impact of their behavior. This acknowledgment helps validate the emotions of the injured party and lays the groundwork for healing. It's essential for the apology to be sincere and heartfelt, showing that the person apologizing truly understands the pain they've caused and regrets their actions.

## 2. Accepting responsibility

Accepting responsibility means owning your actions without making excuses or shifting blame. This apology language emphasizes accountability and integrity. When an injured party values the act of accepting responsibility, they appreciate when the person apologizing acknowledges their role in the situation and takes full accountability for their behavior. It's not enough to merely acknowledge that a mistake was made; individuals who value this apology language expect genuine remorse and a commitment to making things right. Taking responsibility requires humility and courage, as it involves admitting fault and being willing to face the consequences of one's actions.

## 3. Making restitution

Making restitution involves taking concrete steps to repair the damage caused by your actions. This apology language focuses on actions rather than words. When an injured party values the act of making restitution, they expect tangible efforts to right the wrongs committed. This may include offering to fix or replace what was damaged, reimbursing for any losses incurred, or taking proactive measures to rectify the situation. Making restitution demonstrates sincerity and commitment to making amends, showing the other person that their well-being and satisfaction are paramount. It's about actively demonstrating care and concern for the person who was wronged and taking responsibility for the consequences of your actions.

## 4. Genuinely repenting

Genuine repentance goes beyond surface-level apologies and involves a sincere commitment to changing your behavior. This apology language also focuses on actions rather than words. When an injured party values genuine repentance, they expect to see concrete evidence that the person apologizing is genuinely remorseful and willing to make efforts to avoid repeating the same mistakes in the future. This may involve seeking counseling, undergoing personal growth and development, or implementing strategies to prevent similar situations from arising. Genuine repentance requires self-awareness, humility, and a willingness to confront and address your shortcomings. It's about demonstrating through actions that you are committed to becoming a better person and repairing the damage caused by your actions.

## 5. Requesting forgiveness

Requesting forgiveness involves directly asking for forgiveness from the person who was wronged. This apology language focuses on closure and reconciliation. When an injured party values being asked for forgiveness, they find validation and healing in extending forgiveness to the other person and moving forward with the relationship. This step is crucial for both parties to experience closure and move past the hurt and resentment caused by the offense. Requesting forgiveness requires vulnerability and humility, as it involves admitting fault and asking for mercy and understanding from the injured party. It's about acknowledging the pain caused and expressing a genuine desire to restore the relationship to a place of trust and mutual respect.

## Determining the right apology language to use

At some point in almost every relationship, someone might have a bad day, be upset, and feel hurt or offended. You may want to clean it up, but here's the challenge—how do you know someone's apology language to actually get the apology right, so it lands for *them*? First, start with Chapman and Thomas's apology language quiz to understand your own apology language. Then share it with others you are in relationship with. Alternatively, you can ask the person you've harmed what sort of apology they need. See the Resources section for more information.

If that doesn't work, Chapman and Thomas recommend a fool-proof approach—use them all! They recommend taking a few minutes and writing, typing, or dictating a short apology that uses all of the five apology languages. It can be short and to the point, but touch on all of them. The point is of course your intention—to make amends and to heal the relationship. Even *if* your apology is not perfect, most people can still feel and hear your sincerity. I have found this to work so well across all types of relationships, even with total strangers. If you have time, script it out, read it once or twice, get it in your heart, and ask the injured party if it's an appropriate time to make amends or to apologize. I have found that people are indeed more than open to hear an apology.

Even if they do not accept any responsibility for their part of the misunderstanding or miscommunication, *you* can at least "clean up your side of the street," as they say in the recovery world, and do your part to make amends that work, promote empathy, enable understanding, and heal relationships.

## Be Joyful

During the divorce process, I chose to hire a KonMari Consultant to clear my belongings and tidy things up. It was hard work, yet enlivening to go through everything I own and get rid of anything that did not bring me joy! After I completed this process, I felt an uplevel of vibrational energy in my home and in my being. I felt the stagnant energy leave and create space for more vibrant uplifting energy—vitality!

In scripture we are taught that:

"(Wo)Men are that they might have Joy"![24]

In fact, Russel M. Nelson has said that "we are to have joy, not guilt trips."[25]

How often do we get stuck in the endless "doing" list that we forget to stop and smell the roses; that is, to stop and do something that brings us joy? How often do you feel guilty that you *are* stopping to have some fun or cultivate joy? Do you even remember what brings you joy?

When we are young, we are able to tap into joy so quickly. However, as we age and take on the responsibilities of adulthood, we seem to put those joy-enhancing activities on the shelf. There are some who believe that life should include a lot of suffering. For others, they just have not given themselves *permission* to have joy. What is blocking your joy?

Did you know that joy can enhance your vitality? Dr. Ernest Rossi writes that deeply meaningful experiences that incorporate "fascination, mysteriousness and meaningful experiences" signal an unusually strong occurrence of gene expression, brain plasticity (developing new neuronal pathways), and mind/body healing.[26]

Additionally, research shows that joyful people have less chance of a heart attack, healthier blood pressure, lower cholesterol, and can manage their weight better.

Here are ten more reasons why you may want to incorporate more joy into your life:[27]

- Joy feels good
- Joy makes you laugh more and this releases powerful endorphins of happiness
- Joy is healthy
- Joy makes joy
- Joy motivates
- Joy inspires interest

- Joy creates connection
- Joy is freedom
- Joy attracts money
- Joy is your natural state

Even with joy being our natural state, there is little research on it. There is perhaps even some mystery around joy.[28] Pamela Ebstyne King, Ph.D. stated:

> "I have observed that many people have an enduring and underlying sense of something that is deeper than the emotion of happiness, and I have come to describe this as joy. In my study of joy, I have also noticed that joy is more complex than a feeling or an emotion. It is something one can practice, cultivate, or make a habit. Consequently, I suggest that joy is most fully understood as a virtue that involves our thoughts, feelings, and actions in response to what matters most in our lives. Thus, joy is an enduring, deep delight in what holds the most significance."

For me, learning new things brings me fascination. Yup, studying DNA and how we can tweak biochemistry with our diet and lifestyle intrigues and empowers me!

Serving others brings me great meaning and joy! Helping change the trajectory of someone's health from a disease state to vitality brings me meaning.

- My family, especially grandkids, light me up!
- Nature lights me up! Learning a new outdoor skill like sailing and surfing light me up!
- Music lights me up! Well, it can actually fill my soul in profound ways.
- Watching the sunset brings me quiet, peaceful joy.
- Soaking my feet in the ocean water or, better yet, bobbing up and down in the waves brings me great joy.

- My little YorkiePoo Gemma brings me delight, giggles, and joy
- Watching the pelicans dive brings me awe and joy
- Dolphins and big ol' manatees make me giggle and bring exquisite joy

Write down a list of what brings you joy. I love the advice of Optimize Coach Brian Johnson:

> "Follow Your Bliss. Not someone else's idea of your bliss. Not what you think should be your bliss. Not what you think would impress the crowd or appease the family. YOUR bliss."

What if you followed your bliss? If Dr. Averill says that we can "learn, practice, cultivate, or make a habit" of joy, then let's do it!

## Consider This

- Look in your life and your relationships and see where you are not free to "give as before."

- Where, or with whom, are you still holding onto negative, low-vibration emotions that you need to let go of?

- To whom do you owe an apology? What apology language do you think you should use?

- Can you create a "floor" to support you in adding joy to your life daily?

- What brings you fascination? What brings you meaning? What lights you up? What makes you giggle? What brings you joy?

*Eighteen*

# Your Daily Vitals

*"Wellness is a connection of paths:*
*knowledge and action."*
~JOSHUA WELCH

Thus far, I have discussed how to implement the Creation Principles of "See," "Say," and "Feel" (in relation to the spiritual, emotional, and mental bodies) to create your Future-Self vision of the new vital you. Now, it's time to put all of this into action and focus on the "Doing" for the health of your physical body.

As I've stated earlier, both women and men put off self-care, and the cost is so high! Women are the life-source for their families. God divinely designed us this way. Yet, when we neglect ourselves, then our ability to be the life-source diminishes. And we are not just hurting ourselves, we are hurting those who love us and need us. For many, our reach can be far greater than just our own four walls.

Let's face it, the world is in great need for power from nurturing feminine energy in all realms. The "Daily Vitals" outlined in this chapter are essential activities that you can do to support yourself and nurture your divine feminine energy and intrinsic life force. You need to fine tune these Daily Vitals to fine tune your impact in the world.

# Breathe

Our breath has a powerful impact on our brains. Your brain uses 20 percent of the oxygen that comes into your body. Your brain needs oxygen to think powerfully and to remain calm.

In his book, *Breath In, Breath Out*,[1] peak performance guru Jim Loehr states:

> "The key to emotional control is breath control. Breath control is the ultimate weapon. It is the simplest, safest, cheapest, most accessible handle there is for mastering emotional control, for recharging the Ideal Performance State in response to problems, for staying in control, for becoming a peak performer. Breath control is the force that leads to the emotional control that leads to the winning feat."

Breathing controls the Autonomic Nervous System (ANS). As a reminder here, the ANS is divided into the Parasympathetic Nervous System (the "Pretty Safe Nervous System") and the Sympathetic Nervous System (the "Survival Nervous System").

Our breath also has a powerful impact on our cardiovascular health. Researchers from Yale University School of Medicine found that meditating three times a week for six weeks improved endothelial (the lining of our vessels from head to toe) function and reduced blood pressure, resting heart rate, and the risk of heart disease.[2]

The problem is, when we are under stress, we tend to take

> *"Breathing control gives man strength, vitality, inspiration and magic power."*
>
> ~ZHUANGZI

shallow breaths and breathe from our shoulder area. That's what we *don't* want to do. We can find ourselves clenching our body. Our chests are clenched, our shoulders are raised, and our necks are tight. This unconscious practice of gripping our breath is impacting our health unknowingly. Learning how to pay attention to our breathing and then regulate it through intentional breathing takes practice, but the payoff is immense in minimizing the effects of stress on our body.

Diaphragmatic breathing is one of the best and simplest ways to initiate the "Pretty Safe Nervous System" response.

## Diaphragmatic breathing

As we move our breaths down our torso, from our neck and shoulders to the lower belly, we start to engage the Parasympathetic Nervous System. Put your hand on your belly and raise your belly as you take an inhale. This is called diaphragmatic breathing. If you're not familiar with the diaphragm, it's a small muscle right below your lungs. If you're breathing "correctly," it will contract and move downward so that your lungs can expand to take in fresh air. Upon exhalation, the opposite happens—it relaxes and slides further up your chest cavity. This technique slows your breathing and decreases your oxygen needs as it strengthens your diaphragm.[3]

## Practice diaphragmatic breathing

1. Begin with one hand over your heart
   and one hand over your belly.
2. Breathe in through your nose and let the air fill your belly. Keep your hands on your heart and belly and observe how the one on your belly moves while the one on your heart should stay the same.
3. Draw your navel in toward your spine as you exhale as if you were blowing out birthday candles.

4. Feel as the hand on your belly slides down to its original position.
5. Repeat these steps three to five times to start, noticing how you feel each time.

Whenever you experience a negative, stressful trigger, then stop, notice, and take some big diaphragmatic breaths. When you are able to take deep belly breaths, you change the biochemistry of your brain and reclaim your sense of calm. That way, you have the power to *create* a response versus a reaction. I promise, *everything* is better when we can slow down and take some deep breaths!

## 4-7-8 breathing technique

This technique, developed by Dr. Andrew Weil, is a variation of pranayama, an ancient yogic technique that helps people relax as it replenishes oxygen in the body. This technique can help you quickly master your emotions and reduce the cortisol cascade of stressful hormones flowing through your body.

1. Allow your lips to gently part.
2. Exhale completely, making a breathy *whoosh* sound as you do.
3. Press your lips together as you silently inhale through the nose for a count of 4 seconds.
4. Hold your breath for a count of 7.
5. Exhale again for a full 8 seconds, making a whooshing sound throughout.
6. Repeat 4 times when you first start. Eventually work up to 8 repetitions.

## Mouth breathing versus nose breathing

If you are a mouth breather, then you are like most people in our society. Nose breathing is more difficult. It takes longer and forces the oxygen through a smaller passage. This is why it's more nourishing.

Mouth breathing is shallow and causes us to over breathe. Here's a quick chemical breakdown of breathing:

1. You inhale oxygen
2. You exhale carbon dioxide ($CO_2$)
3. $CO_2$ is what controls your breathing. When $CO_2$ reaches a certain level, it sends a signal to the brain to inhale and start the cycle again.

The more active we are, the more $CO_2$ is produced. That's why we breathe more when we are running or jumping compared to when we are sitting or resting.

The optimal resting breathing rate is 3.5 to 5 breaths per minute. Mouth breathing requires us to breathe more, typically as much as 18 to 25 breaths per minute. This over-breathing means you will experience a low-grade form of hyperventilation, which upsets the oxygen and $CO_2$ balance. Thus, we end up with too much oxygen in our body, and we exhale too much carbon dioxide at the same time. Surprise, surprise—we trigger the fight or flight SNS. If you struggle with feeling anxiety, chances are you're over-breathing and experiencing low-grade hyperventilation.

## Hydrate

Obviously, we need to hydrate! That's why it's among the Daily Vitals. It is one of the easiest things you can do to feel good.

Water is critical for every biochemical process in our bodies. Our body is made up of 50 to 75

*"Water is the most neglected nutrient in your diet, but one of the most vital."*

~JULIA CHILD

percent water, depending on our age. Water brings life! Think of the energy that comes from water in our world, and you can probably imagine the impact of water in our cells and tissues. Look at how many great cities and civilizations are built around bodies of water. It's critical for our survival. It also:

- Helps regulate our internal body temperature
- Allows us to sweat and perspire, which facilitates detoxification
- Helps us breathe and perform respiration
- Allows us to produce saliva and digestive enzymes
- Helps us metabolize macronutrients (fats, carbohydrates, and proteins) from the foods we eat and turn them into usable "fuel"
- Helps our muscles contract
- Makes up part of our blood that carries oxygen throughout our bodies
- Helps flush away waste and toxins through urination and bowel movements
- Lubricates our joints and acts as a shock-absorber for our major organs, including the brain, spinal cord, and heart

In the best-selling book *Quench*,[4] Dr. Dana Cohen and Gina Bria share amazing insights from indigenous tribes about adequate hydration. Dr. Cohen states that, "There is no better way of getting structured water but by eating plants." Just think, we can get *double* the benefit by eating our green veggies—phytonutrients *and* water! Try eating a cucumber salad for lunch, and you may find that your afternoon fatigue diminishes. Dr. Cohen reinforces that "Afternoon fatigue is more likely dehydration."

Online sites, such as Consumer Reports, often use a rating system of "good," better," or "best" for products. The choice for any one of these categories may be based upon budget, time, and end results. You know …the ol' *bang for the buck*. So, I am going to share some tips as "good," "better," and "best" when it comes to the choices you make about your hydration.

Good

Avoid dehydrating drinks like coffee, tea, soda, and alcohol.

Drink 16 oz. when you first get up in the morning. This will jump start your cellular function and increase your chance of enjoying optimal wellness. Increase your water intake to 50 percent of your weight in ounces.  If you must have a cup of caffeine to kick start your morning or afternoon, a good rule of thumb is to have at least two cups of water to offset the dehydrating effects of that cup of coffee.

Better

Avoid water in soft plastics (they contain bisphenol A or BPAs that are toxic). The BPA in those bottles will clog up your endocrine system and cell receptors and create a lot of symptoms, including impacting your waistline, your mood, your memory, your sex drive, your cancer risks, and so much more! A simple floor that I do each day is fill up my stainless-steel water bottles early in the morning and keep them by me during the day. I take one in the car, keep one on my desk, and even keep one at my bedside at night.

Best

Do the "good" and "better," as listed above, and filter your water. Purchase the best water filter that you can get, both for drinking and bathing water. If you can't afford one for bathing, at least improve what you drink by eliminating the toxins and chlorine. You can try:

- Alkaline water
- Structured water

- Bless your water
- Add Himalayan salt to your water
- Eat veggies like cucumbers and celery
- Hydrogen Water – there are considerable benefits to Hydrogen water, including increased anti-inflammatory properties, increased anti-oxidant properties, increased energy, slows down the aging process, and improves recovery after workouts. You can find various filters on the internet. Whole house units can be very expensive, yet single bottles can be less than $100. See my resource section for more info.

# Nourish

Following a diet versus nourishing your body are two very different concepts. I've witnessed many diet trends in the last 40 to 50 years, and I even took part in some of them. I remember the days of the Hollywood cabbage soup diet, the grapefruit diet, the lemonade diet, the explosion of the Atkins diet, the low-fat high-carb diet, and the high-fat, low-carb Ketogenic diet. Let's not forget vegetarian, vegan, and plant based. Did I miss one you've tried?

*"Those who think they have no time for healthy eating will sooner or later have to find time for illness."*

~EDWARD STANLEY

Your body has millions of biochemical reactions going on all the time. The biochemistry involved to run this high-tech wonder called your body is mind-boggling, and it is fueled by proper nutrition.

Over the years, the quality of our food supply has diminished significantly. As mentioned earlier, Dr. Lusting's *Metabolical*[5] book clearly uncovers the tragedy of our modern, processed food in the SAD and MAD diets. Most of our major health conditions are indeed a reflection of the defects in our metabolism caused by eating inferior processed food.

In fact, now the recommendation is to eat seven to nine fruits and veggies per day. It used to be five to seven to get adequate nutrition. Because so much of our food has been processed and is biochemically dead by the time we eat it, experts say that many of us are now *"overweight yet undernourished."* The adage "You are what you eat" has evolved to "You are what you absorb." This brings us back to the importance of a healthy gut microbiome so we can optimally digest our food. Without proper digestion we cannot absorb the important micronutrients that are incredibly necessary cofactors in the many biochemical processes in our body. If you are lacking the vitality that *you* Crave, carefully evaluate the food or fuel that you are putting into your body.

This startling quote from Michael Pollan is spot on.

> "The two things are synergistic, the health care crisis
> and the food crisis. Right now, to a large extent, the food
> industry's biggest product is patients for the health care
> industry, and we have to break that."
>
> ~Michael Pollan

Indeed, we have to do something to break that!

> "…we now know that food is information, not just
> calories, and that it can upgrade your biologic software.
> The majority of chronic disease is primarily a food borne
> illness. We ate ourselves into this problem and we have to
> eat ourselves out of it."
>
> ~Mark Hyman, M.D.

## Bio-individualized nutrition

After studying DNA testing for several years, I strongly feel that our way of eating needs to be bio-individualized. There is no "one-size-fits-all" diet. But whatever you do eat, stopping when you're 80 percent full is the best way to optimize your DNA. Again, so perfectly stated by Michael Pollan:

> "If it came from a plant, eat it;
> if it was made in a plant, don't."
> ~Michael Pollan

## Best food choices to optimize *your* DNA

Your best food choices (vs. diet) should be bio-individualized to optimize *your* DNA. For instance, if you have the ApoE4 gene that puts you at a higher risk for Alzheimer's disease, it would be optimal to limit dairy and high fat food. If you have genes that put you at a higher risk for diabetes, such as ACSL1 or WFA1, then you will want to exert special attention to control the timing of your carbohydrates and be certain that you include optimal fiber, whole foods, and exercise.

Even if you choose not to do a DNA test, you can easily look at your family medical history and surmise that you *might* be at higher risk for certain diseases and choose wisely from there. This has been my approach since I was a teenager. When I did finally get my DNA test done, it confirmed many of the food choices that I had already made, and enabled me to refine other things that I was not aware of (i.e., some challenges with gluten).

## Best food choices to optimize *anyone's* DNA

- Fiber, greens, protein, and healthy fats (i.e. avocados) at every meal. Then you can add from that to create the rest of your meal.

- Lots of vegetables and fruits, raw and organic, if at all possible
- Cruciferous vegetables daily and enjoy sprouts as well (especially broccoli)
- Grass-fed, wild caught, free range meats and fish
- Anti-inflammatory foods (if you follow the top three recommendations, you'll be on your way)
- Stop eating when you're 80 percent full

I have included several books on nutrition in my Recommended Readings section that can support you in choosing the best plan for you. If you really want to get bio-individualized answers, then I recommend a DNA test. You can see information in my Resources section.

## The top three foods to reduce/avoid

If you want to restore your nourishment by eating food that is natural, whole, and happy as possible, minimize these "foods":

### Sugars, white flours, and refined carbohydrates

These ingredients are the hallmarks of "The Modern American Diet (MAD)." In fact, "Over the course of the past two hundred years, we've increased our sugar intake by 3,000 percent. This is the single biggest change to the human diet since the invention of fire."

> "Of course, it's also a lot easier to slap a health claim on a box of sugary cereal than on a potato or carrot, with the perverse result that the most healthful foods in the supermarket sit there quietly in the produce section, silent as stroke victims, while a few aisles over, the Cocoa Puffs and Lucky Charms are screaming about their newfound whole-grain goodness."
> ~Michael Pollan

## Vegetable oils

We've discussed "Frankenwheat" and "Frankenbelly," as coined by William Davis M.D., in his seminal book *Wheat Belly* released in early 2022. Well, another major cause of dis-ease from our MAD and SAD diets are from an imbalance of toxic Omega 6 oils to healthy Omega 3 oils. I call those toxic Omega 6 Transfat Oils "FrankenFats" or "FrankenOils."

Transfats are the bad oils that are primarily made up of hy-drogenated oils. In the process of hydrogenation, these oils are chemically changed by manufacturers to increase the shelf life of products. In the process, they alter the oil structure making it much more dangerous! In fact, these "Frankenfats" are known to dramatically increase the risk of cardiovascular disease—both heart attack and brain attack (stroke) as well as certain cancers.[6]

These "Frankenfats" are most commonly found in commercial baked good (donuts, cookies, crackers, croissants, pizza dough, etc.) and in other processed foods such as microwave popcorn, non-dairy creamers, margarine, and shortening. I remember the ad from years ago that said, "Everything is better with Blue Bonnet on it." Well, as it turns out, everything is made more toxic with these Frankenfats on it—or *in* it!

*"Don't eat anything incapable of rotting."*

~MICHAEL POLLAN

Years ago, I did an experiment with some hamburger buns that someone brought to my home for a potluck BBQ. I left them in the pantry for four months, and they sat there for four months without growing mold! Four months! That's the power of trans fats and other fake ingredients in our processed foods.

While the U.S. Food and Drug Administration (FDA) now requires all food companies to phase out artificial trans fats (or partially hydrogenated oils), many products containing trans fats still sit on store shelves and may do so for years, as the distribution process cycles through. So, watch out for trans fats in the products you buy.

### Factory farmed animals, fish, and dairy

Another critical aspect of the MAD diet that is most detrimental to our brain functioning is the factory farming of cows, pigs, chickens, and even fish. Not only are these creatures pumped full of antibiotics and hormones to promote their growth, but they feed on an unnatural diet of grain, which leaves their flesh deficient in many of the very fats and nutrients our brains have required from animals since the dawn of humankind. Unfortunately, adding to the sugar, carbs, and Frankenfats, these antibiotics lead to a growing waistline and a shrinking brain. This is hardly the picture of vitality! Additionally, adding to the adage of "You are what you eat" is "You are what *they* eat, too!"

## Fuel your vitality with smoothies

One of the ways I've found to get the nourishment I need is by eating raw organic fruits and veggies in the form of a green smoothie. You can add all kinds of yummy, nutritious ingredients to your blender to create an amazing nutritious drink.

Be careful not to include a large dose of carbs and high sugary fruit in the morning. This can cause problems for your blood sugar and cortisol balance. I tweak recipes to keep them lower carb and to add a nutrition boost. I delete the frozen bananas and add Hemp, chia seeds, flax seeds, and coconut.

## Read the labels

Is what you are putting in your body whole, real food? Or it is filled with junk that will cause *Metabolical* disease?

It is much better to pay the grocer for healthy organic whole food, than to pay the doctor to fix a bad diet. We will pay, either way!

## Honor your body

The scriptures teach to honor our bodies; that is, our body temples that hold our spirits. They also warn of evil designs in the latter days that may impact our bodies.

> Behold, verily, thus saith the Lord unto you: In consequence of evils and designs which do and will exist in the hearts of conspiring men in the last days, I have warned you, and forewarn you, by giving unto you this word of wisdom by revelation.[7]

The conspiring designs are not relegated only to substances like alcohol and drugs. The conspiring designs exist also in the food-like substances that we see in our grocery stores and used in restaurants.

I listened to an interview recently with Glenn Livingston, PhD.[8] Dr Livingston is a brilliant psychologist and the former CEO of two consulting firms that provided millions of dollars of research to Fortune 500 clients, many in the food industry. As Dr. Livingston said in his interview, he was basically "working on the dark side" sharing secrets with these big companies about how to market to all of us and increase the likelihood that we would buy their products. He stated that there are numerous toxins that are put in foods with the intent to create addiction. He then related a shocking story about leaving a board meeting of one of the companies that he consulted for. The CEO of the company actually turned to him and said, "The best thing we did for the stocks was to take the money out of the product ingredients and put it into the packaging." In other words, this company is more interested in pleasing its stockholders and making the big bucks versus your health or mine. Remember this!

Many, if not most, manu-factured products contain excitotoxins that hijack your brain and create chemical depen-dency. The whole goal is to get you addicted to their products. Your safest bet is to eat whole, organic food that you make in your own home. If you are going to eat "junk food," at least make it yourself. Homemade ice-cream with organic dairy and monk fruit sweetener is a delight and just as yummy without the toxins.

> *What? know ye not that your body is the temple of the Holy Ghost which is in you, which ye have of God, and ye are not your own? For ye are bought with a price: therefore glorify God in your body, and in your spirit, which are God's.* [9]

## Move

Movement is way more important than exercise. Healthy move-ment is another way that we can honor our body temples.

A regular exercise routine or going to the gym a few days a week is great! However, it's much more important to create a *lifestyle* of movement. Simple things like taking the stairs, doing housework, tending your garden, walking your dog, getting up from your desk every 20 minutes, and parking your car farther from the door are all good examples of incorporating more move-ment throughout your day.

Here's what's amazing. Constant movement throughout the day can actually generate a higher Heart Rate Variability (HRV) score (which is an indication of overall health) than if you went to the gym for an hour. Thus, the concentrated effort at the gym may not actually be as healthy for your body as simply moving all day long.

## Movement improves cardiovascular system flow

Movement enhances the development of collateral circulation in the heart, increases V02 max and the efficiency of how the heart and lungs function, and reduces blood pressure.[10,11,12]

> "What may be reassuring, however, is to think of exercise as an insurance policy that may offer both short- and long-term protection for your heart. A single exercise session may protect the cardiovascular system for two to three hours, the authors postulate. In essence, you're training your heart to be more resilient," says Dr. Wasfy.[13]

Additionally, movement supports weight control, helps strengthen muscles, helps to quit smoking, can reverse or slow diabetes, lowers stress, and reduces inflammation. All of these indirect measures also dramatically improve heart health.[14,15,16]

## Movement improves lymph flow

Lymph nodes provide antigens to purify fluids that can contain anything from allergens to cancer cells. That fluid is called lymph. There is more lymph in your body than blood, but there is no pump for lymph. If lymph doesn't move out of small lymph nodes through their ducts into the kidneys and liver, it backs up like a clogged sewer line. So, what's the solution? Movement, especially jumping on a minitrampoline or rebounder.[17]

I mentioned the rebounder in depth in Chapter 12, yet I want to emphasize again that this is an important form of movement when vitality and longevity are you goal. The minitrampoline or rebounder that I recommend is the Cellerciser brand. See my Resources section for more information.

Each time you bounce you increase the gravitational pull on your lymph. You're getting low level "Gs"or increased gravitational pulls similar to what you feel from sudden changes of vehicular speed or carnival rides. With intense walking or rebounding, the "Gs" are in vertical alignment with your body and its lymph system.

Improved lymph flow supports your immune system to produce cells that help you prevent and even fight disease. Additionally, improved lymph flow or drainage supports breast health by filtering out toxins that may increase our risk of breast disease.

## Movement improves hormone function and hormone metabolism

When you move it stimulates the hormones of metabolism—testosterone, growth hormone, adrenaline, ghrelin, epinephrine, and even the hormones of hunger. More importantly, movement impacts sex hormone *metabolism*—eliminating the bad estrogens in the body.

One of the biggest risks that we have today for hormone-related cancers is poor hormone metabolism, as we discussed in Chapter 14. Movement dramatically helps detox the bad foreign estrogens called "xenoestrogens" by improving hormone metabolism through the healthy metabolism pathways.

Here's a study[18] that reveals how movement influences that metabolism. Young women were randomized into two groups—those that did 30 minutes of moderate to vigorous aerobic exercise five days a week for sixteen weeks, or those that led a usually sedentary lifestyle control group. Urine samples were taken to assess their estrogen metabolites to examine the effects of exercise on 2-OH,16-OH, and 4-OH pathways. The women who were using predominantly the healthy 2-OH metabolism had a significant increase in aerobic fitness and a significant decrease in body percent fat. More importantly, the healthy 2-OH levels increase significantly ($p=0.043$) in the experimental exercise group and decreased in the sedentary control groups. Let me translate this for you. The women who had a regular exercise program had healthy hormone metabolism, a significant decrease in body percent fat, and resultant decreased risk for hormone-related cancers. This is clear physiological evidence on a cellular level of why exercise is so important!

The authors stated the conclusion of the study was "our results suggest that changes in premenopausal estrogen metabolism may be a mechanism by which increased physical activity lowers breast cancer risk." Did you get that? Movement reduces breast cancer risk and supports breast health!

## Movement improves mood

In her book *The Joy of Movement*,[19] author Kelly McGonigal shares this inspiring statistic:

"In the United States, daily physical activity—as captured by an accelerometer —is correlated with a sense of purpose in life. Real-time tracking also shows that people are happier during moments when they are physically active than when they are sedentary. And on days when people are more active than their usual, they report greater satisfaction with their lives."

Other experiments in the U.S. and UK have forced moderately active adults to become sedentary for a short time, only to watch their well-being wither. Regular exercisers who replace physical activity with a sedentary activity for two weeks become more anxious, tired, and hostile. When adults are randomly assigned to reduce their daily step count, 88 percent become more depressed! Within one week of becoming more sedentary, they report a 31 percent decline in life satisfaction!

> "The average daily step count required to induce feelings of anxiety and depression and decrease satisfaction with life is 5,649. The typical American takes 4,774 steps per day. Across the globe, the average is 4,961."
>
> ~Kelly McGonigal

Read that again. The average American only walks 4,774 steps per day, and research shows that the threshold when anxiety and depression begin to rear their ugly heads is 5,649 steps. Isn't that shocking? We wonder why so many people are depressed! Anti-depressants are prescribed at an alarming rate globally. The western world had the market size valued at $15,651,000 in 2020 and is expected to be over $21,004,800 by 2030![20]

What if our best medicine was simply to add nourishing food and regular movement? I think one of the greatest benefits of movement is connecting our bodies to our spirits. That is why movement uplifts your mood and provides joy.

## Tips to move more

Optimize Coach Brian Johnson teaches a lot about movement. He coined the acronym "OTM" which means Opportunities to Move. To support our OTMs, Johnson created this powerful formula to help us consistently get more movement.

**1: One deep breath** or sun salutation

**10: Pick an exercise that will get your heart rate up and do 10 of them.** Turning from side-to-side at the waist, jumping jacks, cat/cows, stepping in place, jump rope, or anything else that you prefer to get your heart rate elevated. Personally, I like jumping on my rebounder when I need a boost of productivity and brain power.

**100:** Can you **repeat the above set of 10, 10 times throughout the day**? You may need to create new creation patterns to do this, but it can be fun.

**1,000: Move your body at least every 1,000 seconds.** This is every 16 minutes (16.20 *to be exact*). Physiological imbalances, including changes to insulin and blood sugar can begin in as early as 20 minutes of stationary time![21,22]

**25: Move for a consistent 25 minutes each day.** This does *not* need to be aggressive "exercise." A nice walk outside may be optimal. Besides, fresh air and sunshine naturally magnify the effects of the movement.

## What's your energy level?

Consider the continuum of Yin to Yang energy and determine which end you are typically on. Are you a fast-paced kind of person, with a lot of natural movement and a high stress life? If so, adding some milder Yin supportive movement like Yoga or Thai Chi may be the best movement for you during the day. On the other hand, if you are low on the energy spectrum, a good, fast-paced walk or jumping jacks may be the best fit.

Some may wonder how to move if you are in a long meeting or riding on a plane or have a long daily commute? There are little things you can still do to have some movement. Can you bend your knees? Wiggle your toes? Move at the waist? Flex your feet, stretch your calves, roll your neck? I've noticed on recent plane rides that they now have a seated Yoga stretch routine that passengers can do. If you are creative, you can move.

Remember, the more you incorporate movement that you love, the more you will enjoy it. Additionally, if you're an extrovert and would prefer exercising with company, then invite a friend to join you or call someone while you're on your walk. If you prefer a meditative quiet walk, great. If you prefer listening to music of a podcast, "Just Do It" as Nike says, and get moving!

## What exercise is best for you?

We all have preferences for exercise. I feel that the best exercise is the exercise that you enjoy doing and will incorporate into your life on a regular basis. However, our genetics can determine which form of exercise may be a better option for us, thus the reason that I love people to get their DNA tested. For some, a 50:50 ratio of aerobics to strength training is good; for others a 75:25 ratio may be better. I found with my DNA testing that I clear lactic acid a bit slower, so adding more Epsom salt baths is also helpful. Additionally, I need to pay special attention to stretching due to my SNPs. Below, I share some of the benefits of various forms of exercise to help you see that a well-rounded approach is the best for optimizing your vitality and longevity.

### Aerobics

The importance of aerobic exercise cannot be overstated. From cardiovascular health and weight management to mental well-being and respiratory function, engaging in regular aerobic activities contributes significantly to a holistic approach to fitness and overall vitality. As I stated above, one of the greatest benefits of aerobic exercise is the impact on hormone metabolism, which lowers your risk for all hormone-related cancers, including breast, ovarian, uterine, and prostate. Incorporating aerobic exercise into your routine fosters a healthier and more balanced lifestyle, with far-reaching benefits for both the body and the mind.

I encourage my clients to find some form of aerobics that they love to do.

- Walking
- Running
- Biking
- Kayaking or paddle sports
- Dancing
- Pickleball or Tennis (especially if it's singles)
- Etc.

Here's the deal, we may not enjoy "exercise" but, you are caring for your body so that your body will care for you for many years to come. Remember compound interest from Chapter 3?

### Strength training

Strength training, also known as resistance training or weightlifting, is a crucial component of maintaining vitality, especially as individuals age. As the body undergoes natural physiological changes over time, including a gradual decline in muscle mass and bone density, strength training emerges as a powerful countermeasure with a multitude of benefits.

*"The only way to keep your health is to eat what you don't want, drink what you don't like, and do what you'd rather not."*

~MARK TWAIN

Sarcopenia, the age-related loss of muscle mass, can lead to decreased strength, mobility, and overall functional ability. Regular strength training helps mitigate this loss by stimulating muscle protein synthesis, promoting muscle growth, and improving muscle quality. This is particularly important for maintaining independence and the ability to perform daily activities with ease.

Strength training also supports bone health, which becomes increasingly important as people age. Weight-bearing exercises, such as lifting weights, create stress on bones, prompting them to adapt and become denser. This can help prevent osteoporosis and reduce the risk of fractures, providing a foundation for skeletal strength and durability in the later years of life.

Strength training also has notable metabolic benefits. As individuals age, there is a tendency for metabolism to slow down, leading to weight gain and a decline in overall metabolic health. Strength training helps counteract this by elevating the resting metabolic rate from increased muscle mass. This can contribute to better weight management and improved metabolic function.

Strength training is also linked to enhanced joint health and flexibility. Engaging in resistance exercises supports the development of strong connective tissues around joints, reducing the risk of injuries and promoting joint stability. Improved flexibility and range of motion contribute to better overall mobility, making it easier for you to engage in various activities and maintain an active lifestyle.

Strength training also has profound effects on cognitive function. Recent research[23] suggests a positive correlation between resistance training and cognitive abilities, including memory and executive function. The mental engagement required during strength training, as individuals focus on proper form and technique, contributes to the overall cognitive benefits of this type of exercise.

Obviously, incorporating regular strength training into your routine can significantly enhance overall well-being and contribute to a more active, independent, and fulfilling lifestyle in the later years of life. I encourage my clients to do strength training at least two to three times a week. Going to a gym or using weights is not necessary. You can do "full body" strength or resistance workouts with simple bands or even doing body weight exercises, like squats, lunches, and even yoga as a form of full body strength.

## Pilates

Pilates is a powerful and holistic form of fitness that transcends the traditional boundaries of exercise by promoting overall well-being and vitality. At its core, Pilates focuses on developing a strong and flexible body through a series of controlled movements that engage both the body and mind. The method was developed by Joseph Pilates in the early 20th century and has since gained widespread recognition for its transformative effects.

I have been practicing Pilates for over twenty-five years. I love it so much that years ago, when some stocks I invested in were closing early, and I got a nice-sized check in the mail, I invested in a Pilates combo unit (both the Cadillac and Reformer in one cool interchangeable piece of equipment). I can tell you, it was one of the best investments in my life, as it has changed my level of strength and helped heal significant issues with my musculoskeletal frame.

One of the key reasons Pilates is so effective in supporting vitality is its emphasis on core strength and stability. The exercises target the deep muscles of the core—the abdominals, back, and pelvic floor—leading to improved posture and balance. This not only enhances physical performance, but also helps prevent injuries and contributes to a strong foundation for everyday activities.

Pilates incorporates a range of dynamic movements that promote lengthening and stretching of muscles, reducing stiffness and increasing overall flexibility. Improved flexibility is crucial for maintaining joint health, reducing the risk of injuries, and promoting a sense of ease and fluidity in movement.

Pilates is also a low-impact exercise that can be adapted to suit individuals of all fitness levels. The focus on controlled, precise movements allows for a mindful and meditative experience, fostering a connection between the body and mind. This mind-body awareness cultivated through Pilates can have positive effects on mental well-being by reducing stress and promoting a sense of relaxation and rejuvenation. In fact, I truly love the exercise of my brain almost as much as my body as I focus on each exercise.

In essence, Pilates stands out as a powerful form of fitness that goes beyond the superficial aspects of physical appearance. By promoting core strength, flexibility, and a mind-body connection, Pilates supports overall vitality, helping individuals not only look good but also feel strong, agile, and energized in their daily lives. As my coach Joel Crosby states, "If you want to resist gravity, do Pilates."

## Yoga

Flexibility—the ability of joints and muscles to move through their full range of motion—is crucial for performing daily activities with ease, preventing injuries, and preserving a high quality of life. Maintaining flexibility is paramount for overall health and well-being, especially as individuals age. As the body naturally undergoes changes over time, including a gradual reduction in muscle elasticity and joint mobility, incorporating activities like yoga into a regular routine becomes increasingly important.

Yoga, with its emphasis on gentle, controlled movements and stretching exercises, is a powerful tool for promoting and preserving flexibility in individuals of all ages. The various poses and stretches in yoga promote flexibility by elongating muscles and improving joint mobility. This can help counteract the stiffness and reduced range of motion that often accompany aging, allowing individuals to maintain their ability to move freely and comfortably.

The gentle, controlled movements in yoga improves joint health by encouraging the synovial fluid within joints to circulate, providing lubrication and nourishment to the cartilage. This helps prevent stiffness, reduces the risk of arthritis, and supports overall joint function. Improved joint flexibility also contributes to better balance and coordination, reducing the likelihood of falls and related injuries.

Yoga also has a profound impact on mental well-being. The mind-body connection cultivated through yoga practices, including breath control and mindfulness, promotes relaxation and stress reduction. As stress and tension are known contributors to physical stiffness, the mental benefits of yoga indirectly support flexibility by creating a more relaxed and supple body.

Regular practice of yoga can also alleviate the discomfort associated with common age-related conditions such as lower back pain and arthritis. The gentle stretches and poses in yoga help relieve tension in the muscles and improve circulation, contributing to pain relief and enhancing overall comfort.

The combination of physical and mental benefits makes yoga a well-rounded approach to preserving and improving flexibility. By incorporating yoga into a regular routine, you can enjoy increased joint mobility, reduced stiffness, and a greater sense of overall well-being.

Personally, I love that there are so many forms of yoga, suited to almost anyone, whether it's more of a calming, soothing, relaxing routine to prepare you for sleep, or a vigorous from of Ashtanga power flow yoga, you can find something to suit your needs and preference.

## Sleep

Sleep can be elusive to too many, maybe even you. In the U.S. alone, according to estimates, 50 million to 70 million[24] people have ongoing sleep disturbances. Sleep disorders affect 39 percent to 47 percent of perimenopausal women and 35 percent to 60 percent of postmenopausal women.[25] Up to 75 percent of older adults experience symptoms of insomnia.[26]

Those are some staggering statistics! Insufficient sleep is prevalent globally and across all age groups,[27] is considered to be a public health epidemic that is often unrecognized and under-reported, and has significantly high economic costs.

A clinical paper by Vijay Kumar Chattu, M.D. of Trindad and Tobago, titled "The Global Problem of Insufficient Sleep and Its Serious Public Health Implications"[28] states that "insufficient sleep leads to derailment of body systems." If that's the case, why have we been so lackadaisical with our sleep? Or worse, why is it considered a badge of honor when we plow through our days and nights without sufficient sleep?

Do you have days when you feel you're running on empty? For women, one of *the* most important "tank fillers" or priceless commodities is *good, quality, sleep.* However, sleep is often the very first thing that we choose to sacrifice.

## The toll of sleep deprivation

Renowned double board-certified sleep expert, W. Chris Winter, M.D., summarizes in his book, *The Sleep Solution – Why Your Sleep Is Broken and How to Fix It,*[29] the many reasons why we need to take our sleep seriously.

### Sleep and your brain

I'll bet I'm not alone in recalling a day of incredible brain fog because of a poor night's sleep. Sleep deprivation impacts our attention, cognition, working memory, mood, and productivity.[30] In recent years, we have begun to understand more about the power of the sleep and its impact on the brain.

Earlier (in Chapter 8), I discussed the importance of the lymph system in detoxifying the body. In 2015, scientists discovered that the brain has its own drainage system called the glymphatic system. The glymphatic system is 60 percent more productive when we are asleep. Even more so, apparently, when we sleep on our side.

Scientists discovered that one of the main waste products that the glymphatic system eliminates is amyloid beta, the protein that accumulates in the brain of Alzheimer's patients. It's the ApoE4 gene that increases the risk of Alzheimer's disease by ten- to thirty-fold over those who do not possess it. If you knew that you had the ApoE4 gene and that there was something simple you could do to reduce your risk, would you do it? It turns out that sleep does just that.

A 2013 study in JAMA followed 698[31] older participants in a large community-based study. Sleep was assessed as part of the study. While 98 of the participants developed Alzheimer's, those that slept better had the ability to reduce the impact of the ApoE4 gene on disease severity. Simply sleeping better delayed the onset and severity of the disease for those at higher risk!

Even if you do not have the ApoE4 gene, the toll of sleep deprivation on your brain is intense.[32,33]

## Sleep and obesity

Did you know that sleeping less than six hours and staying up after midnight have been linked to obesity?[34] Ghrelin, a hormone that acts on the brain to promote hunger, is produced in the gut. Ghrelin makes us crave all of the produced, sugar-laden foods in the center aisles of the store or in fast-food establishments. Studies have shown[35] that as sleep decreases, Ghrelin increases, increasing the likelihood of overeating and obesity.[36,37]

### Sleep and your heart

As Dr. Winter states in his book, sleep deprivation is more damaging to the heart than any other organ. It increases blood pressure and increases the risk for a heart attack, heart failure, and stroke.[38] Sleep deprivation has also been associated with abnormal heart rhythms such as atrial fibrillation.[39,40]

### Sleep and your mood

How does sleep deprivation impact your mood or the mood of your family members? What about your co-workers? Poor sleep has been linked to greater depression and anxiety. Interestingly, one study showed[41] that interrupted sleep actually had a more profound effect on mood than shorter-duration sleep. No wonder some of the residents whom I worked with during years of those long days and nights in big medical centers were moody (me included). Their sleep was interrupted all night long!

### Sleep and cancer

While there is evidence that poor sleep quality is linked to an increased risk of cancers (prostate, oral, nasal, and colorectal), it is the risk of breast cancer that seems to be the strongest. In fact, shift work revealed a significant decline[42] in the function of the immune system and a subsequent rise in breast cancer.

### Sleep and your immune system

Perhaps you were raised by your mother or grandmother telling you that "if you didn't get to bed, you're going to catch a cold." Well, they were right. Our immune system and our sleep are inextricably linked. Not only is sleep deprivation associated with generalized immune depression,[43] but researchers in Taipei, Taiwan,[44] revealed that sleep deprivation is a significant risk factor for developing auto-immune symptoms.

## Sleep and your hormones

Our sleep-wake cycles, also known as circadian rhythms, trigger nearly every hormone in our body to release. Sleep deprivation impacts glucose metabolism, but also impacts sex hormones, too. In fact, sleep deprivation can impact[45] hormone synthesis/secretion, follicle formation, ovulation, fertilization, implantation, and menstruation.

Our sleep-wake cycles trigger nearly every hormone in our body to release. Sara Gottfried, M.D., a clinical assistant professor in the Department of Integrative Medicine at Thomas Jefferson University states:

> "When ignored, poor sleep will make you fall down a
> hormonal flight of stairs … That's true whether you're
> 30, 50 or 70."

If your brain is not functioning properly, then your endocrine (hormone) system can't function properly either. Sleep impacts our hormones, and improper hormone balance impacts our sleep. In fact, "Whenever we chronically disrupt sleep in quantity and quality, we disturb this balance and leave the door open to medical problems," says Dr. Abhinav Singh, M.D., medical director of the Indiana Sleep Center.

If your endocrine system gets out of whack, this can create an imbalance in many hormones, including your sex hormones and cortisol levels, which in turn puts demands on your adrenal glands, messes with your appetite and hunger signals, and in the long run even impacts your waistline!

## Get better sleep

Are you convinced that making sleep a priority is imperative to vitality? If you want to improve your sleep, here's some simple sleep hygiene or sleep rituals that I have shared with my clients for years. I invite you to implement these to improve *your* sleep—they work!

- Use your bed for *only* two things—sleep and sex.
- Sleep in a dark room. If you can't get it dark, use an eye mask over your eyes.
- Keep the room cool—less than 65 degrees is best.
- Limit the noise, or have some "white noise," like a fan.
- Use ear plugs if you have a noisy bed partner.
- Avoid heavy meals before bed.
- Avoid sugary or caffeinated drinks before bed.
- Turn off the Wi-Fi when you go to bed.
- Keep electronic equipment away from you.
- Keep your cell phone plugged in another room.
- Keep your screens on night mode at least two hours before your bedtime.
- Wear blue-light blocking glasses after dusk.
- Create a "digital sunset" by turning off devices an hour before sleep.
- Keep the same sleep-wake schedule every day, including on the weekend.
- If you do sleep poorly, limit your sugar intake the following day to compensate for disrupted insulin levels.
- Invest in a high-quality mattress—preferably one that is organic and not filled with toxic VOCs or mold. Personally, I use an organic Dulop latex mattress. See the Resources section for more information.

I also recommend taking the "Chronotype Quiz" quiz by Michael Breus, PhD. Dr. Breus is a world-renowned sleep expert, and his quiz can help you discover your personal *chronotype*, so that you actually start sleeping at the time that is optimal for you!

Although this list is not exhaustive and there are many other factors that contribute to sleep disturbances, you can at least start here to improve your chance of getting *restorative* sleep. That is the most important takeaway for your health and vitality.

Congratulations on making it this far. Clearly, you're the kind of person that is serious about creating greater vitality. I offer support in various ways to meet your specific needs, from bio-individualized private coaching to group coaching, keynote speaking and corporate events. For more information, start here: https://LoriFinlay.com/Start

## Consider This

- How many ounces of water are you drinking each day?

- How can you improve your hydration?

- What toxic foods do you need to eliminate from your diet?

- What's a simple "floor" that you can incorporate to support healthy eating?

- What are your favorite ways to move?

- How do these various movements improve your focus and mood throughout the day?

- What's a simple "floor" that you can incorporate to support healthy movement throughout your day?

- What activities are you doing in bed that may be sabotaging your sleep?

- What's a simple "floor" that you can incorporate to support restorative sleep?

# Section 8

## Closing Thoughts

# *Nineteen*

# Become Your Future-Self

*"The ways you have learned to survive may not
be the ways you wish to continue to live."*
~Dr. Thema Bryant-Davis

You have a far greater capacity to Create the Vitality You Crave than you may have ever imagined. Beginning with your Future-Self in mind, you can consciously create—with each thought and every habit—what you *become*.

Take me, for example.

Two years ago, I was wrapping up what I thought was my first draft of this book. But then my life took that fateful turn into a divorce without warning. At that time, my Future-Self included enjoying retirement with my ex-husband, playing with my grandkids, serving God, completing this book, and seeing where God wanted to lead me in teaching people how to tap into their own divine healing powers.

During the difficult divorce days, weeks, and months, I had to reign in those other dreams. My Future-Self was focused on completing that huge transition with grace and ensuring that I was optimizing my own health spiritually, emotionally, mentally, and physically. During that journey, I laid a new foundation for my ultimate healing, by practicing the potent creator habits I've described in this book and by wisely curating my relationship circles.

Now, as I have grown stronger and better trust my intuition, my healing is more pronounced and creates new possibilities for me to experience new levels of vitality every day. In fact, my recent lab data revealed the proof. My White Blood Count (WBC) that was once 2.8 (when I was called "chemo girl") is now 8.4! Just two years ago, I was elated when it was 5.4. Because of consistent efforts to heal, my immune function is better than it has been in thirty years. Additionally, my Phenotypic (biological) age is now nine years younger than my chronological age. Biohacking works!

My enhanced vitality includes greater peace and calm as well as long nights of deep, restorative sleep. As such, my greater physical stamina now fuels greater opportunities to share my passion and hard-earned wisdom as well as the drive and cognitive function to make a greater difference in this world! I'm stunned by the many doors that have opened for me to spread the word about Epigenetics, functional medicine, and creating vitality, including guest spots on TV, podcasts, and international radio shows; speaking at major corporations; and yes, publishing this book.

The spiritual planting of seeds a few years back are now sprouting because of the Creation Principles of See, Say, Feel, and Do. I'm living proof that we can use these principles in every area of our lives to create a life of freedom, vitality, and passion.

The renowned Dr. Lissa Rankin, in her book *Mind Over Medicine*,[1] proved her hypothesis that life vitality, disease prevention, and optimized remission of disease depends upon:

- Healthy relationships
- A healthy, meaningful way to spend your days
- A healthy, fully expressed creative life
- A healthy spiritual life
- A healthy sexual life
- A healthy financial life
- A healthy environment

- A healthy mental and emotional life
- A healthy support system that supports physical health of the body, such as good nutrition, regular exercise, adequate sleep, and avoidance of unhealthy addictions

My earnest prayer in writing this book has been that it would enlighten and empower you to access your divine healing capacity. Moreover, I pray that the tools I have shared will enhance your ability to create new practices and habits that will restore the vitality you have long been craving.

In Chapter 3, I discussed the law of compound interest. That law is real, and it works upon our physical health with as much precision as it does upon our fiscal health. Truly, "out of small things proceedeth that which is great."[2] Each tiny "floor" you honor and every small habit you create compounds its goodness upon itself to positively impact your health. The small things *do* matter. Your *self*care *is* sacred and expands your embodied presence as a life source in your cherished relationships. Again, as Lalah Delia stated, "Vibrating higher is how you take your power back—on all levels." The Law of Compound Interest in your relationships directly impacts your vitality as well. "The right people bring your soul medicine"[3] is a maxim worth exploring.

## Take Full Ownership of Your Vitality

This is your time. "Quit making excuses. Instead, take EXTREME Ownership of EVERYTHING in your life," states retired Navy Seal Jocko Willink.

In the first place, you are your own soul's number one right person. You are your body's highest authority. Reject the medical gaslighting that says your symptoms are "within normal limits" (WNL) or easily explained away as being "typical for a person your age." Trust *your* gut. Listen to *your* intuition. You're the one in your body—you know when your body is well and vital, and you know when it is not.

Second, your medical provider needs to be as interested as you are in restoring your wellness. Be tenacious in finding the right medical partner, one who values your specialized insight into the world of living in *your* body. You deserve that.

Third, the relationships you nurture either bless or rob your vitality. I learned by hard experience with the Law of Compound Interest that years of people-pleasing, over-functioning, and rescuing depleted me. Honoring myself and loving others with clear, decisive boundaries blessed all of my relationships—whether they were relationships I kept or relationships I released—and helped bring my whole being into vital, healthy balance.

Finally, I invite you to a new wellness model: nourish yourself spiritually, emotionally, mentally, and physically—whether, in the farm-acy of your elevated thoughts or the farm-acy of your clean, whole-foods stocked fridge. Make new "floors" to enhance how you breathe, what you eat, how you move, and when you sleep. Cleanse and detox every area of your life that drags on your vitality, whether environmental, parasitical, or fungal. Release unhealthy, unstable, dysfunctional relationships; these bring trauma and stress to your entire being, throwing all of your systems out of alignment. Magnify your efforts and expand your daily joy with a gratitude journal.

I echo renowned cardiovascular surgery pioneer, Russell M. Nelson, who currently presides as a prophet to over 17 million people.

> "There are specific ways in which we can likely improve. One is the way we treat our bodies. I stand in awe of the miracle of the human body. It is a magnificent creation,

essential to our gradual ascent toward our ultimate
divine potential ..."[4]

Your body is the temple of your spirit.

You *do* have choice.

You have choice Every. Single. Day.

You have choice Every. Single. Bite.

You are a powerful creator who can optimize your health and the expression of your unique DNA.

Vitality is the manifestation of *beingness*. It is part of our becoming. Dallin H. Oaks eloquently teaches that, "We're not just given the opportunity to learn something new. We're given the opportunity to *become* something new. Becoming something new goes far beyond affirming belief in certain ideas. Becoming is a process of conversion, which entails a profound change in nature."[5] My prayer is that my work enlightens and motivates you, perhaps even sparking a conversion process; you indeed can unlock your innate healing powers to create change in your day-to-day life. You have the power to become a person who experiences vitality.

From my heart to yours, may you choose to joyfully Create the Vitality You Crave.

# References

**INTRODUCTION**

1  Bowen, D., Poole, S., White, M., et al., (2021, February 15). "The Role of Stress in Breast Cancer Incidence: Risk Factors, Interventions, and Directions for the Future." *Int J Environ Res Public Health.* 2021 Feb 15;18(4):1871.

**CHAPTER TWO: DYSFUNCTIONAL VERSUS FUNCTIONAL MEDICINE**

1  Lustig, Robert, MD, MSL, *Metabolical: The Lure and the Lies of Processed Food, Nutrition, and Modern Medicine* (Harper, May 2021).

2  Goldstein, S. R. (2023, March 7). "Progesterone." *Healthy Women.*

3  Asi, N., Mohammed, K., Hydour, Q. et al., "Progesterone vs. synthetic progestins and the risk of breast cancer: a systematic review and meta-analysis" *Syst Rev* 5: 121.

4  Lewis, P., (2019, October 14). "HRT and breast cancer risk." *BMJ Publishing Group Ltd.*

5  Santen, R., (2003, November). "Risk of breast cancer with progestins: Critical assessment of current data." *Steroids.* 2003 Nov. 68(10-13):953-64.

6  Rossouw, J. (1996, December 1). "Estrogens for prevention of coronary heart disease. putting the brakes on the bandwagon." *Circulation,* 94(11):2982-5.

7  Bluming, A., MD, and Tavris, C., PhD, *Estrogen Matters,* p.331 (Little Brown Spark, 2018).

8  Parker-Pope, T., *The Hormone Decision* p.14 (Rodale Books, 2007).

9  Langer, R., (2017, April). "The evidence base for HRT: What can we believe?," *Climacteric* April, 20(2):91-96.

10  Lobo, R., (2013, May 01). "Where Are We 10 Years After the Women's Health Initiative?" *The Journal of Clinical Endocrinology & Metabolism.* Pages 1771–1780. Volume 98.

11  Newton, K., LaCroix, A., Leveille, S., Rutter, C., Keenan, N., & Anderson, L., (1997, August). "Women's beliefs and decisions about hormone replacement therapy." *J of Women's Health.* 6(4):459-65.

12  Henderson, B.E., Pagnini-Hill, A., Ross, RK, "Decreased Mortality in users of Estrogen Replacement Therapy" (1991). Arch Intern Med. 151:75–78.

13  Anand, P., Kunnumakkara, A., Sundaram, C., Harikuma, K., Tharakan, S., Lai, O., Sung, B., & Aggarwal, B., (2008, September). "Cancer is a preventable disease that requires major lifestyle changes." *Epub, 2008,* 25(9):2097-116.

**CHAPTER FOUR: GETTING TO THE ROOT CAUSE**

1  Uchtdorf, D., (2010, October 01). "Of Things That Matter Most."

2  *The Doctrine and Covenants of The Church of Jesus Christ of Latter-day Saints.* Salt Lake City, UT: The Church of Jesus Christ of Latter-day Saints, 1981. Section 130:20-21.

**CHAPTER FIVE: MAKE THE MOST OF YOUR EPIGENETIC POWER**

1  Lipton, Bruce, Dr., (2019, August 20). Unity North Atlanta Church, 4255 Sandy Plains Road Marietta, GA.

2  Ibid.

3  Smith, Margaret, Williams, Sue, *Gene Genius* (Harlequin, 2015).

4 Lynch, Ben, Dr., *Dirty Genes* (Harper One, 2020).

5 Willett, W. (2002, April 26). "Balancing life-style and genomics research for disease prevention." *Science*, 2002, 296(5568):695-8.

6 Lipton, Bruce, Dr., The Biology of Belief: Unleashing the Power of Consciousness, Matter and Miracles, pg. 72 (Efinito, 2022).

7 Ibid.

8 Richards, R. Aziz, N., Bick, D., et al. (2015, May). "Do all gene variants affect health and development?" *Medline Plus*.

9 Moore, D., Shenk, D., (2017, January). "What are the different ways a genetic condition can be inherited?" *National Library of Medicine*.

10 *The Book of Mormon*. Trans. Joseph Smith, Jr. Salt Lake City, UT: The Church of Jesus Christ of Latter-day Saints, 1981, 2nd Nephi 2:27.

## CHAPTER SIX: USE THE POWER OF CREATION PRINCIPLES

1 *The Pearl of Great Price of The Church of Jesus Christ of Latter-day Saints*. Salt Lake City, UT: Moses 2:3-4.

2 *The Book of Mormon*. Trans. Joseph Smith, Jr. Salt Lake City, UT: The Church of Jesus Christ of Latter-day Saints, 1981, 2nd Nephi 2:13-14.

3 Cobb, et al., (1959, May 28). "NEJM."

4 Dimond, E., Kittle, C., & Crockett, J. (1960, April). "Comparison of internal mammary artery ligation and sham operation for angina pectoris." *Am J. Cardiol.* (1960) April; 5:483-6.

5 Siegel, Bernie, Love, Medicine & Miracles: Lessons Learned about Self-Healing from a Surgeon's Experience with Exceptional Patients, p. 47 (Harper Paperbacks, 1990).

## CHAPTER EIGHT: CLEANSE YOUR BODY

1 Bush, Z., (2017. March 23). "Dr. Masaru Emoto and Water Consciousness." *The Wellness Enterprise*.

2 Spanne, A., (2022, February 15). "What are PFAS?," *Environmental Health News*.

3 Landi, S., (2000, October). "Mammalian class theta GST and differential susceptibility to carcinogens: a review." *Science Direct*. Volume 463, Issue 3, Pages 247-283.

4 Laukkanen, T., Khan, H., Zaccardi, F., & Laukkanen, J., (2015, April). "Association between sauna bathing and fatal cardiovascular and all-cause mortality events." JAMA *Internal Med*. 2015 April;175(4):542-8.

5 Kwik, Jim, *Limitless Expanded Edition: Upgrade Your Brain, Learn Anything Faster, and Unlock Your Exceptional Life* (Hay House, 2023).

## CHAPTER NINE: CLEANSE YOUR ENVIRONMENT

1 (2022, December) "Air pollution," *World Health Organization*.

2 Mercola, Joseph, M.D., EMF*D: 5G, Wi-Fi & Cell Phones: Hidden Harms and How to Protect (Hay House, 2020).

3 Kelly, E., (2019, October). "The International EMF Scientist Appeal serves as a credible and influential voice from EMF (electromagnetic field) scientists who are urgently calling upon the United Nations and its sub-organizations, the WHO and UNEP, and all U.N. Member States, for greater health protection on EMF exposure." *EMF Scientist*.

## CHAPTER TEN: CLEANSE YOUR MENTAL AND EMOTIONAL BODIES

1 Kwik, Jim, Limitless Expanded Edition: Upgrade Your Brain, Learn Anything Faster, and Unlock Your Exceptional Life (Hay House, 2023).

2 Truman, Karol, *Feelings Buried Alive Never Die* (Olympus Distributing, 1995).

3  Brennan, Barbara, *Hands of Light* (Pleiades Books, 1987).
4  Rosenburg, Ross, PhD, *The Human Magnet Syndrome: The Codependent Narcissist Trap"* (Independent, 2022).

## CHAPTER ELEVEN: BOOST YOUR CELLULAR POWER AND COMMUNICATION

1  Wu G, Fang YZ, Yang S, Lupton J R, Turner N D, Glutathione Metabolism and Its Implications for Health, J. Nutr. 2004, Mar;134(3): 489-92.
2  Townsend, D.M., Tew, K.D., Tapiero, H., "The Importance of Glutathione in Human Disease" *Biomed Pharacother,* 2003, May-Jun; 57 (3-4): 145-55.
3  Roberts, J. C.; Charyulu, R. L.; Zera, R. T.; Nagasawa, H.T. (1992). "Protection Against Acetaminophen Hepatotoxicity by Ribose-Cysteine (RibCys)." *Pharmacology & Toxicology,* 70, 281-285.
4  Sabbatinelli, et al., "Ubiquinol Ameliorates Endothelial Dysfunction in Subjects," *Nutrients,* 2020 12, 1098.
5  Schemizer, C., et al., "Functions of Coenzyme Q-10 in inflammation and gene expression," *BioFactors,* 2008.
6  Babacg et al, 2015.
7  Mitchell, H., Hamilton, T., Steggerda, F., Bean, H., (1945, May 1). "The chemical composition of the adult human body and its bearing on the biochemistry of growth." *Journal of Biological Chemistry.* Volume 158, Issue 3. Pages 625-637.
8  Grimsley, R., (2022, November 11). "Hysterectomy: N W H N." *National Women's Health Network.*

## CHAPTER TWELVE: BIOHACKS FOR CELLULAR HEALTH

1  Sinatra, S., "Electric Nutrition: The Surprising Health and Healing Benefits of Biological Grounding (Earthing)." *Altern Ther Health Med,* 2017 Sept;23(5)8-16.
2  Menigoz, W., Latz, T., Ely, R., Kamei, C., Melvin, G., & Sinatra, D., "Integrative and lifestyle medicine strategies should include earthing (grounding): Review of Research Evidence and Clinical Observations." *Explore* (NY). 2020 May-Jun;16(3):152-160.
3  Yap, J., Tai, Y., Fröhlich, J., Fong, C., Yin, J., Foo, Z., Ramanan, S., Beyer, C., Toh, S., Casarosa, M., Bharathy, N., Kala, M., Egli, M., Taneja, R., Lee, C., & Franco-Obregón, A., "Ambient and supplemental magnetic fields promote myogenesis via a trpc1-mitochondrial axis: Evidence of a magnetic mitohormetic mechanics." *FASEB J.* 2019 Nov;33(11):12853-12872.
4  Tabrah, F., Hoffmeier, M., Gilbert, F., Batkin, S., & Bassett, C., "Bone density changes in osteoporosis-prone women exposed to pulsed electromagnetic fields (PEMFs)." *J Bone Miner Res.* 1990 May;5(5):437-42.
5  Li, Y., Li, L., et al., "Enhancing cartilage repair with optimised supramolecular hydrogel-based scaffold and pulsed electromagnetic field." *Bioact Mater.* 2022 Oct 12;22:312-324.
6  Cugusi, L., Manca, A., & Serpe, R., "Effects of a mini-trampoline rebounding exercise program on functional parameters, body composition and quality of life in overweight women." *J Sports Med Phys Fitness.* 2018 Mar;58(3):287-294.
7  Sukkeaw, W., Kritpet, T., & Bunyaratavej, N., "A comparison between the effects of aerobic dance training on mini-trampoline and hard wooden surface on bone resorption, health-related physical fitness, balance, and foot plantar pressure in Thai working women." *J Med Assoc Thai.* 2015 Sep;98 Suppl 8:S58-64.
8  Scrivens, D., (2012, June 8). "Rebounding: Good for the Lymph System." *Well Being Journal.* Vol. 17, No. 3.
9  Cogoli, A., Valluchi, M., Reck, J., Müller, M., Briegleb, W., Cordt, I., & Michel, C., "Human lymphocyte activation is depressed at low-G and enhanced at high-G." *Physiologist.* 1979 Dec;22(6):S29-30.

10 Cogoli, A., "Changes observed in lymphocyte behavior during gravitational unloading." *ASGSB Bull.* 1991 Jul;4(2):107-15.

11 Cho, K.-H., Jung, S.-H., Choi, M.-S., Jung, Y.-J., Lee, C.-G., & Choi, N.-C., "Effect of water filtration infrared-A (WIRA) sauna on inorganic ions excreted through sweat from the human body." *Environ Sci Pollut Res Int.* 2023 Feb;30(7):18260-18267.

12 Sobajima, M., Nozawa, T., Ihori, H., & Shida, T., "Repeated sauna therapy improves myocardial perfusion in patients with chronically occluded coronary artery-related ischemia." *Int J Cardiol.* 2013 Jul 15;167(1):237-43.

13 Beever, R., (2009, July). "Far-infrared saunas for treatment of cardiovascular risk factors: Summary of published evidence." *Can Fam Physician.* 2009 Jul;55(7):691-6.

14 Hussain J., Cohen M., "Clinical Effects of Regular Dry Sauna Bathing: A Systematic Review." *Evid Based Complement Alternat Med.* 2018 Apr 24;2018:1857413.

15 Cleveland Clinic, (2024, March 19). "BRRR! what to know about cold plunges." *Cleveland Clinic.*

16 Aloian, A., (2023, July 7). "8 cold plunge benefits for physical, mental health from experts." *Women's Health.*

17 Gu, Y., Yu, J., Lum, L., & Lee, R. "Tissue engineering and stem cell therapy for myocardial repair." *Front Biosci.* 2007 Sep 1;12:5157-65.

18 Drapeau, Christian, *Cracking the Stem Cell Code: 3rd Edition* (Golden Swan Press, 2021).

19 Chang L., Fan W., Pan X., Zhu X., (2022, April 20). "Stem cells to reverse aging." *Chin Med J (Engl).* 2022 Apr 20;135(8):901-910.

20 Brunet A., Goodell M., Rando T., "Aging and rejuvenation of tissue stem cells and their niches." *Nat Rev Mol Cell Biol.* 2023 Jan;24(1):45-62.

21 Naik S., Larsen S., Cowley C., Fuchs E., "Two to tango: dialogue between immunity and stem cells in health and disease." *Cell.* 2018 Nov 1;175(4):908-920.

22 Nowacki M., Kloskowski T., Pietkun K., et al. (2017, December 31). "The use of stem cells in aesthetic dermatology and plastic surgery procedures. A compact review of experimental and clinical applications." *Postepy Dermatol Alergol.* 2017 Dec;34(6):526-534.

23 Galiè M., Covi V., Tabaracci G., Malatesta M., (2019, August 17). "The Role of Nrf2 in the Antioxidant Cellular Response to Medical Ozone Exposure." *Int J Mol Sci.* 2019 Aug 17;20(16):4009.

24 (2023, February 24) "What Is Ozone Therapy?," *Holtorf Medical Group.*

25 Serra M., Baeza-Noci J., Abdala C., Luvisotto M., Berto C., Anzolin A., (2023 April 15). "Clinical effectiveness of medical ozone therapy in COVID-19: the evidence and gaps map." *Med Gas Res.* 2023 Oct-Dec;13(4):172-180.

26 Konig, B., Lahodny, J., (2022, July 21). "Ozone high dose therapy (OHT) improves mitochondrial bioenergetics in peripheral blood mononuclear cells." *Translational Medicine Communications.*

## CHAPTER THIRTEEN: BALANCE YOUR GUT-BRAIN CONNECTION

1 Carabotti, M., Scirocco, A., Maselli, M. A., & Severi, C., (2015). The gut-brain axis: interactions between enteric microbiota, central and enteric nervous systems. *Annals of Gastroenterology,* 28(2), 203-209.

2 Mayer, E. A., (2011). "Gut feelings: the emerging biology of gut-brain communication." *Nature Reviews Neuroscience,* 12(8), 453-466.

3 Foster, J. A., & McVey Neufeld, K. A., (2013). "Gut–brain axis: how the microbiome influences anxiety and depression." *Trends in neurosciences,* 36(5), 305-312.

4 Robertson, R., PhD., (2023, April 03). "How Does Your Gut Microbiome Impact Your Overall Health?" *Healthline.*

5 DeVos Willem, Tilg Herbert, et al., *Gut Microbiome and Health: Mechanistic insights,* BMJ, Vol, 71, (5).

6  Davis, William, *Super Gut: A Four-Week Plan to Reprogram Your Microbiome, Restore Health, and Lose Weight* (Hachette Go, 2022).
7  Saffouri, G., Shields-Cutler, R., Chen, J., et al., "Small intestinal microbial dysbiosis underlies symptoms associated with functional gastrointestinal disorders." *Nat Commun.* 2019 May 1;10(1):2012.
8  Ogunrinola, G., Oyewale, J., Oshamika, O., Olasehinde, G., (2020, June 12). "The Human Microbiome and Its Impacts on Health." *Int J Microbiol.* 2020 Jun 12;2020:8045646.
9  Mahud R., Akter S., et al., "Impact of Gut Microbiome on Skin Health: Gut-Skin axis observed through the lense of therapeutics. Gut Microbes, 14 (1); 2022.
10  Singh, R., Chang, H., Yan, D., et al., "Influence of diet on the gut microbiome and implications for human health." *J Transl Med.* 2017 Apr 8;15(1):73.
11  Lerner, A., Benzvi, C., "Let Food Be Thy Medicine": Gluten and Potential Role in Neurodegeneration, Cells, 2021 April; 10 (4):756.
12  Rogers, M., PhD, MS, and Aronoff, D., "The Influence of Nonsteroidal Anti-Inflammatory Drugs on the Gut Microbiome." Clin Microbiol Infect. 2016 Feb;22(2):178.e1-178.e9.
13  Weersma, R., Zhernakova, A., Fu, J., "Interaction between drugs and the gut microbiome." Gut. 2020 Aug;69(8):1510-1519.
14  Freedberg, D., Lebwohl, B., Abrams, J., "The impact of proton pump inhibitors on the human gastrointestinal microbiome." *Clin Lab Med.* 2014 Dec;34(4):771-85. *doi: 10.1016/j.cll.2014.08.008.*
15  Ervin, S., Li, H., Lim, L., Roberts, L., et al., "Gut microbial β-glucuronidases reactivate estrogens as components of the estrobolome that reactivate estrogens." *J Biol Chem.* 2019 Dec 6;294(49):18586-18599.
16  Stockdale, Brenda, *You Can Beat the Odds: The Surprising Factors Behind Chronic Illness and Cancer* (Sentient Publications, 2009)..
17  Yaribeygi, H., Panahi, Y., Sahraei, H., et al., "The impact of stress on body function: A review." EXCLI J. 2017 Jul 21;16:1057-1072.
18  Sivasankaran, S., Pollard-Quintar, S., Sachdea, R., et al., The effect of a six-week program of yoga and meditation on brachial artery reactivity" Do psychosocal interventions affect vascular tone? Clin Cardiol. 2006 Setp; 29 (9): 393-398.
19  Goralczyk-Binkowska, A. et al., "The Microbiota- Gut- Brain Axis in Psychiatric Disorders," *Int. J. Mol. Sci.* 2022, Sept 24; 23 (19): 11245.
20  Fernstrom, J., Effects on the diet and brain neurotransmitters, Metabolism 1977 Feb; 26 (2):207-23.
21  Dauvilliers, Y., Tafti, M., and Landolt, H.P., Catechol-O-methyltransferase, dopamine and sleep-wake regulation, *Sleep Medicine Reviews*, Vol. 22, Aug. 2015, p. 47-53.
22  Sevoz-Couch, C., and Laborde, S., "Heart Rate Variability and slow-paced breathing: when coherenece meets resonance." *Neurosci Biobehav* Rev. 2022 April:135:1-4576.
23  . Paerciavalle, P., Blandinin, M., et al., The role of deep breathing on stress, Neurol Sci. 2017 Mar; 38 (3): 451-458.

## CHAPTER FOURTEEN: BALANCE YOUR HORMONES

1  Toufexis, D., Virarola, M.A., Lara, H., Viau, V., "Stress and the Reproductive Axis," J. *Neuroendocrinol,* 2014, Sep. 26 (9):573-86.
2  Ho, G., Lou, X., Ji, C., et al., "Urinary 2:16 alpha-hydroxyestrone ratio: correlation with serum insulin-like growth factor binding protein-3 and a potential biomarker of breast cancer risk." Ann Acad Med Singap. 1998 Mar;27(2):294-9.
3  Miao, S., Yang, F., Wang, Y., Shao, C., et al., "4-Hydroxy estrogen metabolite, causing genomic instability by attenuating the function of spindle-assembly

checkpoint, can serve as a biomarker for breast cancer." *Am J Transl Res.* 2019 Aug 15;11(8):4992-5007.

4  Cowan, L, D., Gordis, J. A., et al., "Breast Cancer Incidence in Women with a History of Progesterone Deficiency," *Journal of Epidemiology,* Vol. 114, (2), Aug. 1981- pg. 209-217.

5  "EWG's Dirty Dozen and Clean Fifteen," EWG.*org.*

6  "Dirty Dozen," EWG.*org.*

7  Dr. Jenn Simmons, Keeping Abreast Podcast 5:: *The Truth about Estrogen and Breast Cancer with Dr. Tabatha Barber,* July 31, 2023.

8  Ibid.

9  Walter, Z., (2021, April 16). "Women's Hormones: The Safety of Bioidentical Hormone Replacement Therapy." *A4M Medicine Refined.*

10  Shockney, L., (2024, January 17). "BRCA: The Breast Cancer Gene." *National Breast Cancer Foundation.*

11  Ibid.

12  Grey, J., "State of the Evidence: The Connection Between Breast Cancer and The Environment," *Environmental Health* (2017) 16 :94.

13  Cavalieri, E., Chakravarti, D., Guttenplan, J., et al. "Catechol estrogen quinones as initiators of breast and other human cancers: implications for biomarkers of susceptibility and cancer prevention." Biochim Biophys Acta. 2006 Aug;1766(1):63-78.

## CHAPTER FIFTEEN: WHOLE BODY ALIGNMENT

1  Van Der Kolk, MD, Bessel, *The Body Keeps the Score: Brain, Mind, and Body Healing of Trauma* (Viking, 2014).

2  Delia, Lalah, *Vibrate Higher Daily – Live Your Power* (Harper One, 2019).

3  KJV *Bible,* 1st Corin. 3:16.

## CHAPTER SIXTEEN: CREATE YOUR CALM FROM WITHIN

1  Pert, Candace, PhD, *Molecules of Emotion: Why You Feel the Way You Feel* (Scribner, 1997).

2  Surtees, P., Wainwright, N., Luben, R., et al., "Psychological distress, major depressive disorder, and risk of Stroke." *Neurology.* 2008 Mar 4;70(10):788-94.

3  Lillberg, K., Verkasalo, P., Kaprio, J., "Stressful Life Events and Risk of Breast Cancer in 10,800 Women: a Cohort Study." *Neurology.* 2008 Mar 4;70(10):788-94.

4  Bitman, B., Berk, L., Shannon, M., et al., "Recreational Music - Making modulates the human stress response: a Preliminary individualized gene expression strategy," *Med Sci Monit* 2005 Feb;111(2):BR31-40.

5  Stockdale, Brenda, *You Can Beat the Odds: The Surprising Factors Behind Chronic Illness and Cancer* (Sentient Publications, 2009).

6  Swenson, Richard A., MD, *Margin: Restoring Emotional, Physical, Financial, and Time Reserves to Overloaded Lives* (NavPress, 2004).

7  KVJ *Bible* Philippians 4:13.

8  *The Book of Mormon.* Trans. Joseph Smith, Jr. Salt Lake City, UT: The Church of Jesus Christ of Latter-day Saints, 1981, Mosiah 4:27.

9  KJV *Bible* - 1 Corinthians 3:16.

10  Mitchell, M., Dr. Herbert Benson's Relaxation Response, *Psychology Today,* March 29, 2013.

11  Sivasankara, S., Pollard-Quitner, S., Sachdeva, R., et al., (2006, September). "The effects of a six-week program of yoga and meditation on brachial artery reactivity: do psychosocial interventions affect vascular tone." Cell. 2018 Nov 1;175(4):908-920. 12 - 2 Nephi 2:26.

12 *The Book of Mormon.* Trans. Joseph Smith, Jr. Salt Lake City, UT: The Church of Jesus Christ of Latter-day Saints, 1981, 2 Nephi 2:14, 16, 26.

13 Menter, Jeanette Elizabeth, *You're Not Crazy, You're Codependent: What Everyone Affected by Addiction, Abuse, Trauma or Toxic Shaming Must know to have Peace in Their Lives* (J2 Publishing, 2012).

14 Lipton, Bruce, Dr., "The Biology of Personal Empowerment," Unity Church, Marietta Georgia, Aug. 20th, 2019.

15 Hazlettk, L., I., Moieni, M., Irwin, M. R., et al., "Exploring neural mechanisms of the health benefits of gratitude in women: A randomised controlled trial, *Brain, Behavior and Immunity* Vol. 95, July 2021, P. 444-453.

16 Wang, X. and Song, C., "The impact of gratitude interventions on patients with cardiovascular disease: a systematic review." *Front Psychol.* 2023 Sep 21;14:1243598.

17 Heart Math Institute, Cohen, Dana, Bria, Gina, *Quench* (Hachette, 2018).

18 Redwine, L., Henry, B., Brook L., Pung, M., et al, *Psychom Med* (2016 Jul – Aug.; 78(6):667-76).

19 Dispenza, Joe, Dr., *The Transformational Power of Gratitude Unlimited.*

20 O'Leary, K., & Dockray, S., (2015, March 31). "The effects of two novel gratitude and mindfulness interventions on well-being." *J Altern Complement Med.* 2015 Apr;21(4):243-5.

21 Aknin, L.B., et al., "Positive Feelings reward and promote prosocial behavior," *Current Opinion in Psychology,* Vol. 20, April 2018, p.55-59.

22 Mao, Y., Zhao, J., Xu, Y., & Xiang, Y., "How gratitude inhibits envy: From the perspective of positive psychology." *Psych J.* 2021 Jun;10(3):384-392.

23 *KJV Bible,* James 1:17.

24 Cauble, M.R., Said, I.M., et al, Religion / Spirituality and the Twin Virtues of Humility and Gratitude, *Handbook of Positive Psychology, Religion and Spirituality,* pp 379-393, 18, Nov. 2022.

25 Chowdhury, M.R., "The Neuroscience of Gratitude and the Effects on the Brain," *Positive Pyschology.com* April, 9, 2019.

## CHAPTER SEVENTEEN: BE YOUR BEST *SELF*

1 Kabat-Zinn, Jon, *Full Catastrophe Living: Using the Wisdom of Your Body and Mind to Face Stress, Pain and Illness* (Random House, 1990).

2 Kabat-Zinn, J., Wheeler, E., Light. T., Skillings, S., et al., (1998, September-October). "Influence of a mindfulness meditation-based stress reduction intervention on rats of skin clearing in patients with moderate to severe psoriasis undergoing Phototherapy (UVB) and Photochemotherapy (PUVA)." *Psychosom Med.* 1998 Sep-Oct;60(5):625-32.

3 Tang, Y.Y., Ma, Y. et al, "Central and Autonomic nervous system interaction is altered by short-term mediation." Proceedings of the National Academy of Sciences, 106 (22),8865-8870.

4 Pressman, S.D., Cohen, S., Miller, G.E., Barkin, A, Rabin, B.S., Teranor, J.J., (2005). "Loneliness, social network size and immune response to influenza, vaccination, in college freshman." *Healthy Psychology,* 24/3/0. 297-306.

5 King James Version, The Holy Bible, Luke 23:34.

6 King James Version, The Holy Bible, Mathew 5:38-44.

7 *The Doctrine and Covenants of The Church of Jesus Christ of Latter-Day Saints.* Salt Lake City, UT: The Church of Jesus Christ of Latter-Day Saints, 1981, Section 64:10.

8 King James Version, The Holy Bible, 1st John, 1:8-10.

9 North, J., (1987). "Wrongdoing and Forgiveness." Philosophy 62: 499-508).

10 Miller, C., Grimm, C. (1979). "Personality and Emotional Stress Measurement on Hypertensive Patients with Essential and Secondary hypertension." *International Journal of Nursing Studies.* p.85-93.

11  Diamond, E. (1982). "The Role of Anger and Hostility in Essential Hypertension and Coronary Disease." *Psychology Bulletin* 92: 410-433.

12  Williams, Virginia and Redford, *Anger Kills: Seventeen Strategies for Controlling Hostility That Can Harm Your Health,* Nov. 4, 1998.

13  (2021, November 1). "Forgiveness: Your health depends on it." *Johns Hopkins Medicine.*

14  Almeida, B., Cunha, C. "Time, Resentment, and Forgiveness: Impact on the Well-Being of Older Adults." *Trends in Pyschol.* (2023).

15  "How the Link between Forgiveness and health changes with age," University of Michigan News.

16  The Power of Forgiveness, Mind & Mood, www.Harvard Health.edu, Feb. 12, 2021.

17  Ibid.

18  Enrich, Robert., PhD, *Forgiveness is a Choice – A Step-by-Step Process for Resolving Anger and Restoring Hope* (APA LifeTools, 2001).

19  Faust, J., *The Healing Power of Forgiveness,* (April 2007) Ensign, The Church of Jesus Christ of Latter-Day Saints.

20  Adams, H., (Oct 15, 2006). "After the Tragic Day, a Deeper Respect Among the English Amish." *Sunday News.* p. 1.

21  Tutu, Desmond, Tutu, Mpho, *The Book of Forgiving – The Fourfold Path for Healing Ourselves and Our World,* (Harper One, 2014).

22  Truman, Karol K., *Feelings Buried Alive Never Die* (Karol K. Truman, Olympus Distributing, 1991 & 2003).

23  Chapman, Gary and Thomas, Jennifer, *The 5 Apology Languages: The Secret to Healthy Relationships* (Northfield Publishing, 2022).

24  *The Book of Mormon,* Trans. Joseph Smith, Jr. Salt Lake City, UT; The Church of Jesus Christ of Latter-Day Saints, 1981, 2nd Nephi, 2:25.

25  Nelson, R., (1995, October). *"Perfection Pending."* The Church of Jesus Christ of Latter-Day Saints.

26  W.W. Norton and Company, (2002, September 17., "The Psychobiology of Gene Expression.")

27  Johnson, T., (2015, November 14). "10 Reasons to Add Joy to Your Life." *Huffpost.*

28  Aten, J., (2020, July 28). "What Is Joy and What Does It Say About Us?" *Psychology Today.*

## CHAPTER EIGHTEEN: YOUR DAILY VITALS

1  Loehr, James E., *Breathe In, Breathe Out: Inhale Energy and Exhale Stress by Guiding and Controlling Your Breathing* (Hanover Square Press, 2022).

2  Sivasankara S., Pollard-Quinter, S., Sachdeva, R. et al., "The effects of a six-week program of yoga and meditation on brachial artery reactivity: do psychosocial interventions affect vascular tone?" *Clin Cardiol.* 2006 Sep;29(9):393-8.

3  Hopper, S., Murray, S., Ferrara, L., et al., "Effectiveness of diaphragmatic breathing for reducing physiological and psychological stress in adults: a quantitative systematic review." *JBI Database System Rev Implement Rep.* 2019 Sep;17(9):1855-1876.

4  Cohen, Dana, M.D., and Bria, Gina, *Quench* (Hachette, 2018).

5  Lustig, Robert, *Metabolical,* The Lure and the Lies of the Processed Food, Nutrition, and Modern Medicine (Harper, 2021).

6  (Feb 23, 2022) "Transfat is double trouble for heart health." Mayo Clinic.

7  *The Doctrine and Covenants of The Church of Jesus Christ of Latter-day Saints.* Salt Lake City, UT: The Church of Jesus Christ of Latter-day Saints, 1981. Section 89:4.

8  Livingston, G. (n.d.), "Glenn Livingston: How to stop overeating and lose weight on the diet of your choice." *Psychology Today.* https://www.psychologytoday.com/us/contributors/glenn-livingston-phd

9   King James Version, *The Holy Bible*, 1 Corinthians 6:19:30.

10  Mobius-Winkler, S., Uhlemann, M., Adams, V., et al., (2016, March 15). "Coronary Collateral Growth Induced by Physical Exercise." *AhaJournals*.

11  Karp, J., (2017, October 25). "3 Workouts to Increase VO2 Max." *Active*.

12  Joyner, M., Coyle, E., (2008, January 01). "Endurance exercise performance: the physiology of champions." *National Center for Biotechnology Information*. 586(1):35-44.

13  Cornelissen, V., Smart, N., "Exercise training for blood pressure: a systematic review and meta-analysis." *J Am Heart Assoc*. 2013 Feb 1;2(1):e004473.

14  "Exercise and the hear.t" *Johns Hopkins Medicine*. 5. (2023, October 10).

15  Laskowski, E., (2022, July 13). "What are the risks of sitting too much?" *Mayo Clinic*.

16  Healy, G., Winkler, E., et al., "Replacing sitting time with standing or stepping: associations with cardiometabolic risk markers." *European Heart Journal*, 36, 39, Oct. 2015.

17  Fassa, P. (2013, October 09). "Using Rebounding and Exercise to Improve Lymph Flow and Feel Better." *Natural Society*.

18  Smith, A., Phipps, W., Thomas, W., Schmitz, K. (2013, May). "The Effects of Aerobic Exercise on Estrogen Metabolism in Healthy Premenopausal Women." *PubMed*. 22(5):756-64.

19  McGonigal, Kelly, *The Joy of Movement: How exercise helps us find happiness, hope, connection and courage*, Avery, March, 2021.

20  "Antidepressant Drugs Market Size, Share, Competitive Landscape and Trend Analysis Report by Product, Depressive Disorder: Global Opportunity Analysis and Industry Forecast, 2021-2030." *Allied Market Research*. (2022 Feb.).

21  Peddie, M., Kessel, C., Bergen, T., et al., "The Effects of Prolonged Sitting, Prolonged standing, and activity breaks, and postprandial glucose and insulin responses: A randomized crossover trial," *PLoS One*, 2021; Jan. 4, 16(1).

22  Dunston, D., Kingwell, B., et al. "Breaking Up Prolonged Sitting Reduces Postprandial Glucose and Insulin Responses," *Diabetes Care*, 2012, May;35 (5):976-83.

23  Broadhouse, K.M., Singh, M.F., et al., "Hippocampal Plasticity unpins long-term cognitive gains from resistance exercise in MCI," *Neuroimage Clinical*, Vol. 25, 2020, 102182.

24  What are Sleep Deprivation and Deficiency? https://www.nhibi.nih.gov/health /sleep-deprivation

25  Joffe, H., Massler, A., Sharkey, K., (2013, August 07). "Evaluation and Management of Sleep Disturbance During the Menopause Transition." *Semin Reprod Med*. 2010 Sep;28(5):404-21.

26  Nguyen V., George T., Brewster G., (2019, October 22). "Insomnia in Older Adults." *Current Geriatrics report*. Volume 8, p. 271-290.

27  Chattu, V., Manzar, D., Kumary, S., et al., (2018, Dec. 20). "The Global Problem of Insufficient Sleep and its Public Health Implications." *Healthcare (Basel)*.

28  Ibid.

29  Winter, Chris, *The Sleep Solution: Why Your Sleep is Broken and How to Fix It* (Berkley, 2017).

30  Krause, A., Simon, E., & Mander, B., (2017, July). "The sleep-deprived human brain." *Nat Rev Neurosci*. 2017 Jul;18(7):404-418.

31  Spira, A., Gamaldo, A., Wu, M., et al., (2013, December). "Self-reported sleep and β-amyloid deposition in community-dwelling older adults". *JAMA Neurology* 70(12):1537-43.

32  Lim, A.P., L. Yu, M. Kowgier, et al., "Sleep Modifies the Relation of ApoE to the risk of Alzheimer's Disease and Neurofibrillary Tangle Pathology," *JAMA, Neurology* 70, no.12 (2013):1544-51.

33  John Hopkins School of Public Health, "Shorter Sleep Duration and Poorer Sleep Quality Linked to Alzheimer's Disease Biomarker," Oct. 12, 2013.

34  Taheri, S., Lin, L., Austin, D., et al., (2004, December). "Short sleep duration is associated with reduced leptin, elevated ghrelin, and increased body mass index." PLoS Med. 2004 Dec;1(3):e62. doi: 10.1371/journal.pmed.0010062.

35  Patel, S. and Hu, F., (2008, March). "Short sleep duration and weight gain: a systematic review." Obesity 16(3):643-53.

36  Hagen, E.W., Starke, S.J., Peppard, P.E., "The Association Between Sleep Duration and Leptin, Ghrelin, and Adiopnectin Among Children and Adolescents." Curr Sleep Medicine Rep 1. 185-194 (2015).

37  Shuailing Liu, Xiya Wang, Qian Zheng, et al., "Sleep Deprivation and Central Appetite Regulation," Nutrients, Dec. 7, 2022.

38  Evabayekha, E. Aiwuyo , H., et al., "Sleep Deprivation Is Associated with Increased Risk of Hypertensive Heart Disease: A Nationwide Population-Based Cohort Study," Cereus, 2022.Dec; 14 (12): e 33005.

39  Kanagala, R., Murali, N., & Friedman, P., et al., (2003, May 27). "Obstructive sleep apnea and the recurrence of Atrial Fibrillation." Circulation 107(20):2589-94.

40  Morovatdar, M., Ebrahimi, N., Rezaee, R., et.al, "Sleep Duration and the Risk of Atrial Fibrillation: a Systemic Review," J. of Atr. Fibrillation, 2019, Apr; 11(6): 2132.

41  Finan, P., Quartana, P., Smith, M., "The Effects of Sleep on the Continuity Disruption on Positive Mood and Sleep Architecture in Healthy Adults," Sleep, 2015, Nov. 1; 38 (11):1735-42.

42  Wang, P., Ren, F., Lin, Y., et al., "Night-shift work, sleep duration, daytime napping and breast cancer risk." Sleep Medicine, April; 16(4):462-8.

43  Garbarino, S., Lanteri, P. Bragazzi, N., et al., "Role of Sleep deprivation in the immune-related disease risk and outcomes," Commun Biol, 2021: 4: 1304.

44  Hsiao, Y., Tseng, T., et al., "Sleep Disorders and Increased Risk of Autoimmune Diseases in Individuals without Sleep Apnea," Sleep, 38, no. 4 (2015) 581-86.

45  Beroukhim, G., Esencan, E., & Seifer, D., (2022, January 18). "Impact of sleep patterns upon female neuroendocrinology and reproductive outcomes: A comprehensive review - reproductive biology and endocrinology." Reprod Biol Endorcinol., 2022, Jan.18; 20 (1):16.

## CHAPTER NINETEEN: BECOME YOUR FUTURE-SELF

1  Rankin, Lissa, Mind Over Medicine (Hay House, Revised 2020).

2  Doctrine and Covenants Section 64 verses 33-34.

3  Delia, Lalah, Vibrating Higher Daily, p.116 (Harper One, 2019).

4  Nelson, R., (April 2019). "We Can Do Better and Be Better." General Conference for the Church of Jesus Christ of Latter-Day Saints.

5  Oaks, D., (Oct. 2000). "The Challenge to Become." General Conference for the Church of Jesus Chris of Latter-Day Saints.

# Resources

If you'd like to tap into my years of expertise that I've distilled into this book and want to use *me* as your personal resource to create lasting changes, then let's start working together, today. https://LoriFinlay.com/start

## Chapter Eight – Cleanse Your Body

### Castor Oil by Queen of the Thrones®

- Queen of the Thrones® is the #1 practitioner-recommended original heatless, less-mess, and reusable Castor Oil Pack Kit designed by a naturopathic doctor to support the relaxed, parasympathetic state.
- This may help naturally support: Liver detox and lymphatic draining and colon cleansing, hormone balance, deep sleep and less stress, constipation and bloating, inflammation and leaky gut.
- This is the product that I personally use and recommend to my clients.

### Cellercizer –rebounder
### Glutathione (GSH) support

I have spent more than 16 years' researching the best forms of Glutathione to support my own health and that of my clients. It took 25 years for nine Ph.Ds. to crack the biochemical code that brought RiboCeine, a magic molecule that helps your body make GSH, to the market. RiboCeine is the only endogenous (made inside the cells) source of Glutathione (GSH) support on the market today, clinically proven in human trials, to raise serum GSH by 26% in all ranges and 64.7% in the 51- to 60-year-old group, in only 4 weeks. To learn more about the science, visit RiboCeine (https://www.ribocysteine.com/).

You can order my favorite products here:

- **Cellgevity ™** (https://lorifinlay.com/glutathione-cellgevity) provides the ultimate in Glutathione enhancement. Cellgevity™ delivers Max's patented ingredient, RiboCeine™, and twelve other essential nutrients that support Glutathione's vital role in removing harmful toxins and neutralizing free radical damage in our body. Cellgevity™ is gluten and melamine free

- **Max One™**, (https://lorifinlay.com/maxone) powered exclusively by Max's RiboCeine™ technology, is the most effective way to deliver the nutrients necessary for your cells to produce Glutathione on demand. MaxOne™ is gluten and melamine free. This product is just one ingredient—Ribocysteine or RiboCeine™ for short. For those that are sensitive to the other GSH boosting ingredients in CellGevity ™, this may be a better choice. Used by Veterinarians as well, I give my little dog one of these every morning.

**Ozone Therapy** (https://www.ozonegenerator.com/)
From pain management to skin rejuvenation and combating infections, ozone therapy offers a versatile and holistic approach to health, empowering the body's innate ability to heal and thrive.

**Sunlighten Infrared Sauna**
(https://lorifinlay.com/sunlight-saunas)
I have personally used Sunlighten for over 17 years. I highly recommended and feel they are the best on the market.

- Infrared Saunas have been shown to clinically improve your health in numerous ways. From weight loss, cleansing, immunity, anti-aging, relaxation, heart health, muscle recovery to just plain ol' relaxation, these saunas are amazing!
- Sunlighten saunas are Patented SoloCarbon 3 in 1 technology, which is the only heater delivering the exact optimal wavelength of near, mid, and far infrared
- 100% solid wood with seamless Magne-Seal technology
- Eco-friendly non-toxic wood, verified low VOC
- Low EMF heating technology

## Chapter Nine – Cleanse Your Environment

**April Aire Indoor Air Filters** (https://shop.aprilaire.com/collections/air-filters) These filters are able to filter particles down to 1 nanogram.

**Environmental Working Group** (https://www.ewg.org/)

**EMF*D Products**
Harmoni Pendant (https://www.harmonipendant.com/)
- Defender Shield phone, computer and tablet cases (https://defendershield.com)
- Young Living Essential Oils (https://wwwyoungliving.com/us/en?enrollerid=1151347)
- Doterra (https://referral.doterra.me/15224576)

IQ-Aire portable filters (https://lorifinlay.com/iq-aire-filters)

**Mead Indoor** (https://meadindoor.com) The air we breathe is 5x more important to our heath than hospitals, physician's, and medications combined. The Mead Indoor Team is personally and passionately committed to the delivery of comprehensive and sustainable indoor environmental solutions that improve lives, wellness, and healing.

**Micro Balance Mold Remediation products** (https://microbalancehealthproducts.com/?rfsn=5808138.c98655) Micro Balance products have been created by Dr. Donald P. Dennis, ENT in Atlanta, GA, USA. Dr. Dennis's pre-med graduate education in microbiology and biochemistry, and his years of working with mold-affected patients make him uniquely qualified to create these cutting edge, lifesaving products. I use them regularly and recommend them to my clients. These proven, non-toxic products, homeopathic formulations, and professional-grade supplements are designed to help you fight mold, whether it's inside your home or your body.

**Ultimatum Bipolar Ionizer** (model UI-AMSD 1100F) (https://ultimatumusa.com)
* Airborne Mitigation system
* Eliminates SARS Covid-2/Covid-19
* Breaks down all viruses' bacteria, mold, VOCs, and odor
* Sanitizes the air and maintains a healthier environment

## Chapter Ten – Cleanse Your Mental and Emotional Bodies

**Brain Spotting** (https://wholetones.com)

**Dance** (https://www.verywellmind.com/dance-therapy-and -eating-disorder-treatment-5094952)

**EDMR** (https://www.emdr.com/what-is-emdr/) EMDR (Eye Movement Desensitization and Reprocessing) is an excellent tool. You can do a search to find a provider near you.

**Essential oils**- I use numerous oils from Young Living (https://lorifinlay.com/young-living-essential-oils) and **DoTerra** (https://store.do-essential-oils.com/?gad_source =1&gclid=CjwKCAjwoa2xBhACEiwA1sb1BDp0T0Mo8pnB bux6tAbP2i3JhFAuADue845Fv6Go0iJK8GroErUWbxo CWJQQAvD_BwE).

**Music** I recommend the Solfeggio music, especially 528 MHz by Whole Tones.

**Yoga** (https://wholetones.com/)

Download Lori's personal SOS list—free "clearing" and "empowerment" tools to help you cleanse and shift your emotional energy anytime you need it. https://CreateTheVitalityYouCrave. com/coaching-resources

## Chapter Eleven – Boost Your Cellular Power and Communication

**Glutathione support**
See Chapter 8 Resource list for detailed information.

**Magnesium** (https://lorifinlay.com/magnesium-breakthrough) harnesses all seven natural magnesium types, free from synthetics, for unmatched potency, promoting better sleep, stress balance, and overall well-being, while also supporting immune function, electrolyte balance, and bone health, challenging the notion that more magnesium equals better health.

## Chapter Twelve – Biohacks for Cellular Health

FREE Biohacking Summary Guide—a quick-reference list of simple, no-cost hacks you can use at home to support your vitality. https://CreateTheVitalityYouCrave.com/biohacking

**Grounding sheets** (https://grounded.com/what-is-earthing)
- **Earthing Collections** (https://www.earthing.com/collections/all?rfsn=4833138.6e8ba8&utm_campaign=4833138.6e8ba8&utm_medium=affiliate&utm_source=refersion)

**Ozone Therapy** (https://www.ozonegenerator.com)
See Chapter 8 Resources list for more information.

**PEMF** (https://www.pulsepemf.com/pemf-machines/)
PEMF, is a revolutionary wellness modality that utilizes soothing Pulsed Electromagnetic Fields to stimulate and exercise the body's cells. PEMF is trusted worldwide to support the body's natural healing and regulating abilities.
- The earth emits a pulsing electromagnetic field at 7.8 hertz. This natural energy field, combined with around 8 million global lightning strikes per day, allows our planet to sustain life. Much like the earth, our bodies are electromagnetic; our brains use electromagnetic signals to communicate with every bodily system.
- Science has proven that if our cells have enough electrical charge, the body will heal itself!

- PEMF is a holistic supplement that infuses the body with natural energy at the cellular level. The body may use that energy to heal and regenerate itself, enhance its natural recovery process, assist with muscle fatigue and discomfort after exercise, increase energy or support relaxation, balance the body's interconnected systems.

**Stem Cell Therapy** (https://lorifinlay.com/stemregen)
Natural ingredients support the release of and migration of 10 million stem cells:

- Stimulates the release of stem cells from the bone marrow
- More stem cells contribute to tissue repair
- Maintain optimal health
- Anti-aging effects

## Chapter Thirteen – Balance Your Hormones

**Hormonal Harmony Quiz**

To bring you clarity and confidence and reignite your power and vitality, I've created a series of hormone quizzes. These quizzes will provide you with valuable insights into potential hormone imbalances that could be the root cause of your symptoms that your doctor may be missing.

You can start with my FREE Estrogen Dominance quiz that will help you navigate the most common of hormone imbalances at https://pages.lorifinlay.com/hormone-quiz

Or

You can take my hormonal harmony assessments which address your sex hormones, adrenal and thyroid hormones too. https://pages.lorifinlay.com/hh-assessments-start

**Consider Supplementation**

If you are interested in gaining access to the best Pharmaceutical grade nutritional products that I recommend to my clients, you can click here and join FullScript.com (https://us.fullscript.com/welcome/womenwisdomwellness/store-start). You can have access to products listed here as well as dozens of personal care products.

- Calcium D- Glucarate
- CellGevity: Click here to order CellGevity and start reducing YOUR toxic load. Once you click on the page, you will see a "welcome" message. Click on the My Account button to create an account to get this amazing product at Wholesale pricing, as my VIP client. Then enjoy the life enhancing benefits!
- DIM Mighty Maca: After drinking green drinks for nearly two decades, Mighty Maca® Plus, is my very favorite!! I use it every day and recommend it to all of my clients. They love it, too!
- Progesterone Cream
- Vitamin B
- Vitamin C
- Vitamin D

## Chapter Sixteen – Be Calm

**Joy Organics** (https://lorifinlay.com/joy-organics) Joy Organics has become a leader in the CBD industry, setting the standards for manufacturing, testing, and quality. Our product development team works tirelessly developing new and improving existing formulas. They have utilized state-of-art technology and sourced the finest ingredients to create products that have imp roved tens of thousands of lives across the country. Joy Organics recently became one of the first major CBD companies to introduce a line of USDA Certified Organic CBD tinctures and jarred salves and remains committed to crafting some of the highest quality products on the market.

## Chapter Seventeen – Be Your Best Self

**DNA Testing**

**Highly Sensitive Persons**
**Your Journal For Life** (https://dayoneapp.com) From DayOne

## To gain access to the entire list of resources in one easy location, scan here.

https://CreateTheVitalityYouCrave.com/book-resources

# Recommended Readings

## Biohacking

- *Boundless: Upgrade Your Brain, Optimize Your Body & Defy Aging* by Ben Greenfield, James Newcomb, et al.
- *Dare to Be 100 99 Steps To A Long, Healthy Life* by Walter M. Bortz II, M.D.
- *Life Force: How New Breakthroughs in Precision Medicine Can Transform the Quality of Your Life & Those You Love* by Tony Robbins, Peter Diamandis, M.D. & Robert Hariri, M.D., Ph.D.
- *How Not to Age: The Scientific Approach to Getting Healthier as You Get Older* by Michael Greger, M.D., FACLM
- *Smarter Not Harder: The Biohacker's Guide to Getting the Body and Mind You Want* by Dave Asprey
- *Young Forever: The Secrets to Living Your Longest, Healthiest Life* by Mark Hyman, M.D.

## Brain Health

- *Change Your Brain, Change Your Life: The Breakthrough Program for Conquering Anxiety, Depression, Obsessiveness, Anger, and Impulsiveness* by Daniel G. Amen, M.D.
- *Unleash The Power of the Female Brain: Supercharging Yours for Better Health, Energy, Mood, Focus, and Sex* by Daniel G. Amen, M.D.
- *Buddha's Brain: The Practical Neuroscience of Happiness, Love & Wisdom* by Rick Hanson, Ph.D.

- *Limitless Expanded Edition: Upgrade Your Brain, Learn Anything Faster, and Unlock Your Exceptional Life* by Jim Kwik
- *The Brain Warrior's Way: Ignite your Energy and Focus, Attack Illness and Aging, Transform Pain into Purpose* by Daniel G. Amen, M.D. and Tana Amen, BSN, RN

## Cleansing

- *Break the Mold: 5 Tools to Conquer Mold and Take Back Your Health* by Dr. Jill Crista
- *EMF*D: 5G, Wi-Fi & Cell Phones: Hidden Harms and How to Protect Yourself* by Dr. Joseph Mercola
- *Mold Warriors: Fighting America's hidden health threat* by Richie C. Shoemaker, M.D., and Patti Schmidt
- *The Detox Solution: The Missing Link to Radiant Health, Abundant Energy, Ideal Weight, and Peace of Mind* by Dr. Patricia Fitzgerald
- *The Life-Changing Magic of Tidying Up: The Japanese Art of Decluttering and Organizing* by Marie Kondo

## Codependency

- *Beyond Codependency and Getting Better All the Time* by Melody Beattie
- *Codependent No More: How to Stop Controlling Others and Start Caring for Yourself* by Melody Beattie
- *You're Not Crazy, You're Codependent: What Everyone Affected by Addiction, Abuse, Trauma, or Toxic Shaming Must Know to Have Peace in Their Lives* by Jeanette Elisabeth Menter

## Creation

- *Living in Your True Identity: Discover, Embrace, and Develop Your Own Divine Nature* by Brooke Snow
- *The Holy Bible*

## Emotions

- *Feelings Buried Alive Never Die …* by Karol K. Truman
- *Molecules of Emotion: Why You Feel the Way You Feel* by Candace B. Pert, Ph.D.
- *Remembering Wholeness: A Handbook for Thriving in the 21st Century* by Carol Tuttle
- *The Emotion Code: How to Release Your Trapped Emotions for Abundant Health, Love, and Happiness* by Dr. Bradley Nelson

## Energy

- *Energy Medicine: Balancing Your Body's Energies for Optimal Health, Joy, and Vitality* by Donna Eden
- *The Hidden Messages in Water* by Masaru Emoto
- *The Cortisol Connection: Why Stress Makes You Fat and Ruins Your Health and What You Can Do About It* by Shawn Talbott, PH.D, FACSM
- *Vibrate Higher Daily: Live Your Power* by Lalah Delia

## Epigenetics

- *Dirty Genes: A Breakthrough Program to Treat the Root Cause of Illness and Optimize Your Health* by Dr. Ben Lynch
- *Gene Genius: Understand Your DNA and Create Your Own Genetic Roadmap to Health and Happiness* by Dr. Margaret Smith
- *Outsmart Your Genes: How Understanding Your DNA Will Empower You to Protect Yourself Against Cancer, Alzheimer's, Heart Disease, Obesity, and Many Other Conditions* by Brandon Colby, MD
- *The Biology of Belief: Unleashing the Power of Consciousness, Matter, and Miracles* by Bruce H. Lipton, PhD
- *The DNA Way: Unlock the Secrets of Your Genes to Reverse Disease, Slow Aging, and Achieve Optimal Wellness* by Kashif Khan

- *Understanding Genomics: How Nutrition, Supplements, and Lifestyle Can Help You Unlock Your Genetic Superpowers* by Marios Michael, D.C., CNS, cFMP

## Environmental

- *Earthing: The Most Important Health Discovery Ever?* by Clinton Ober, Stephen T. Sinatra, M.D., and Martin Zucker
- *EMF*D: 5G, Wi-Fi & Cell Phones: Hidden Harms and How to Protect Yourself* by Dr. Joseph Mercola
- *Mold Warriors: Fighting America's hidden health threat* by Richie C. Shoemaker, M.D., and Patti Schmidt

## Fasting

- *Intuitive Fasting: The Flexible Four-Week Intermittent Fasting Plan to Recharge Your Metabolism and Renew Your Health* by Dr. Will Cole
- *Fast Like a Girl: A Woman's Guide to Using the Healing Power of Fasting to Burn Fat, Boost Energy, and Balance Hormones* by Dr. Mindy Pelz

## Foods

- *Fat for Fuel: A Revolutionary Diet to Combat Cancer, Boost Brain Power, and Increase Your Energy* by Dr. Joseph Mercola
- *Food: What the Heck Should I Eat?* by Mark Hyman M.D.
- *Food Rules: An Eater's Manual* by Michael Pollan
- *Keto-Green 16: The Fat-Burning Power of Ketogenic Eating + The Nourishing Strength of Alkaline Foods = Rapid Weight Loss and Hormone Balance* by Anna Cabeca, DO
- *Keto·tarian – The (Mostly) Plant-Based Plan to Burn Fat, Boost Your Energy, Crush Your Cravings, and Calm Inflammation: A Cookbook* by Dr. Will Cole

- *Metabolical: The Lure and the Lies of the Processed Food, Nutrition, and Modern Medicine* by Robert H. Lustig, MD, MSL
- *Food: What the Heck Should I Cook?* by Mark Hyman, MD
- *The Food Allergy Cure: A New Solution to Food Cravings, Obesity, Depression, Headaches, Arthritis, and Fatigue* by Ellen Cutler M.D.
- *The Inflammation Spectrum: Find Your Food Triggers and Reset Your System* by Dr. Will Cole
- *The Happiness Diet: A Nutritional Prescription for a Sharp Brain, Balanced Mood, and Lean, Energized Body* by Tyler Graham & Drew Ramsey, MD
- *The 150 Healthiest Foods on Earth (Revised Edition): The Surprising, Unbiased Truth about What You Should Eat and Why* by Jonny Bowden, Ph.D, C.N.S.
- *Wheat Belly (Revised and Expanded Edition): Lose the Wheat, Lose the Weight, and Find Your Path to Health* by William Davis, MD

## Forgiveness

- *Forgiveness is a Choice: A Step-by-Step Process for Resolving Anger and Restoring Hope* by Robert D. Enright, PhD
- *Radical Acceptance: Embracing Your Life with the Heart of Buddha* by Tara Brach, Ph.D.
- *Pain is Inevitable, Misery is Optional* by Hyrum W. Smith and Gerreld L. Pulsipher
- *The Book of Forgiving: The Fourfold Path for Healing Ourselves and Our World* by Desmond Tutu and Mpho Tutu

## Habits

- *Atomic Habits: An Easy & Proven Way to Build Good Habits & Break Bad Ones* by James Clear
- *Tiny Habits: The Small Changes that Change Everything* by BJ Fogg, PhD

## Healing

- *Bonds That Make Us Free: Healing Our Relationships, Coming to Ourselves* by C. Terry Warner
- *Breaking the Habit of Being Yourself: How to Lose Your Mind and Create a New One* by Dr. Joe Dispenza
- *It's Just My Nature! A guide to Knowing and Living Your True Nature* by Carol Tuttle
- *Love, Medicine & Miracles: Lessons Learned about Self-Healing from a Surgeon's Experience with Exceptional Patients* by Bernie S. Siegel, M.D.
- *Mind Over Medicine: Scientific Proof that You Can Heal Yourself* by Lissa Rankin, M.D.
- *Remembering Wholeness: A Personal Handbook for Thriving in the 21st Century—20th Anniversary Updated Edition* by Carol Tuttle
- *The Smart Persons Guide to Breast Cancer* – Jennifer Simmons, MD
- *The Thyroid Connection: Why You Feel Tired, Brain-Fogged, and Overweight—and How to Get Your Life Back* by Amy Meyers, MD
- *You Can Beat the Odds: The Surprising Factors Behind Chronic Illness and Cancer* by Brenda Stockdale

## Heart Health

- *Prevent and Reverse Heart Disease: The Revolutionary, Scientifically Proven, Nutrition-Based Cure* by Caldwell B. Esselstyn, Jr., M.D.
- *The HeartMath Solution: The Institute of HeartMath's Revolutionary Program for Engaging the Power of the Heart's Intelligence* by Doc Childre and Howard Martin
- *The Sinatra Solution: Metabolic Cardiology by* Stephan T. Sinatra, M.D., F.A.C.C.

- *Women Are Not Small Men: Life-Saving Strategies for Preventing and Healing Heart Disease in Women* by Nieca Goldberg, M.D.

## Hormones

- *Beyond the Pill: A 30-Day Program to Balance Your Hormones, Reclaim Your Body, and Reverse the Dangerous Side Effects of the Birth Control Pill* by Dr. Jolene Brighten
- *Estrogen Matters: Why Taking Hormones in Menopause Can Improve and Lengthen Women's Lives—Without Raising the Risk of Breast Cancer* by Avrum Bluming, MD, and Carol Tavris, PhD
- *The Hormone Fix: Burn Fat Naturally, Boost Energy, Sleep Better, and Stop Hot Flashes, the Keto-Green Way* by Anna Cabeca, DO, OBGYN, FACOG
- *The Wisdom of Menopause (Revised and Updated): Creating Physical and Emotional Health During the Change* by Christiane Northrup, M.D.
- *Women's Bodies, Women's Wisdom: Creating Physical and Emotional Health and Healing* by Christiane Northrup, M.D.

## Mindfulness

- *At One Ment: Embodying the Fullness of Human-Divinity* by Thomas Wirthlin McConkie
- *Limitless Expanded Edition: Upgrade Your Brain, Learn Anything Faster, and Unlock Your Exceptional Life* by Jim Kwik
- *Full Catastrophe Living: Using the Wisdom of Your Body and Mind to Face Stress, Pain, and Illness* by Jon Kabat-Zinn, Ph.D.
- *Radical Acceptance: Embracing Your Life with the Heart of Buddha* by Tara Brach, Ph.D.

- *The Four Agreements: A Practical Guide to Personal Freedom* by don Miguel Ruiz
- *The God Seed: Probing the Mystery of Spiritual Development* by M. Catherine Thomas
- *The Power of Stillness: Mindful Living for Latter-Day Saints* by Jacob Z. Hess, Carrie L. Skarda, Kyle D. Anderson, and Ty R. Mansfield

## Sleep

- *Lights Out: Sleep, Sugar, and Survival* by T.S. Wiley and Bent Formby, Ph.D.
- *The Sleep Solution: Why Your Sleep is Broken and How to Fix It* by W. Chris Winter, M.D.

## Scripture

- *The Holy Bible*
- *The Book of Mormon: Another Testament of Jesus Christ* by The Church of Jesus Christ of Latter-Day Saints

## Stem Cells

- *Cracking the Stem Cell Code* by Christian Drapeau, MSc.

## Trauma

- *It Didn't Start with You: How Inherited Family Trauma Shapes Who We Are and How to End the Cycle* by Mark Wolynn
- *The Body Keeps the Score: Brain, Mind, and Body in the Healing of Trauma* by Bessel van der Kolk, M.D.

# About the Author

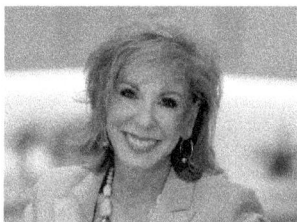

**L**ori Finlay, **MSN, NP, CNS, BCC**, retired nurse practitioner and clinical nurse specialist with over 40 years of experience, is known as the woman's body, mind, and spirit "tune up" specialist. She has helped women all over North America rebalance their hormones, overcome their fear and fatigue, crush their life-sucking symptoms, make sense of their bodies, and recapture their vitality.

Lori has graced stages around the world, from nursing education events, international conventions, and the decks of cruise ships, to appearing on TV segments, podcasts, and radio, including the prestigious Martha Stewart Radio Show. Her extensive expertise in hormones, heart health, Epigenetics, and biohacking, coupled with her personal journey of healing her own body, mind, and spirit, have enabled her unique understanding of the intricacies of women's health through their various stages of life. Lori possesses the ability to distill the sea of information on health and wellness into a clear path for women to invest their time and energy to achieve holistic well-being.

Whether coaching one-on-one, facilitating groups, or working with seminar participants, her clients have lowered their stress, restored their inner calm, rebalanced their hormones, and revitalized their lives. The results are dramatic and life changing.

Lori graduated with her bachelor's in nursing from the University of Utah, a master's degree in nursing from the University of Massachusetts, in Worchester MA, followed by a post-graduate degree as an Adult Nurse Practitioner from the University of Utah. When she's not traveling, Lori lives in St. Petersburg, Florida, with her little Yorkie-Poo named Gemma. Her passions include her family, friends, faith, making a difference, music, and water sports.

Visit her online at:
www.LoriFinlay.com
www.LoriFinlay.com/blog
https://www.Facebook.com/LoriFinlayNPcoaching.com
https://www.instagram.com/LoriFinlayNP.coach